T0113426

BECAUSE EATING RIGHT CAN SAVE YOUR LIFE . . .
CORINNE T. NETZER'S
101 LOW CHOLESTEROL RECIPES

DO YOU KNOW HOW MUCH CHOLESTEROL IS IN THE
FOODS YOU COOK AT HOME?
YOU CAN ELIMINATE THE GUESSWORK WITH DELICIOUS
RECIPES THAT GUARANTEE
A LOW—OR *ZERO*—CHOLESTEROL COUNT AND TELL YOU
THE NUMBER OF MILLIGRAMS IN EVERY SERVING.

SO GIVE YOURSELF PEACE OF MIND *AND* SEE HOW LOW
YOUR CHOLESTEROL INTAKE CAN GET!

◆ Garlic-Dijon Mayonnaise-Style Dressing = .9 mg
◆ Three-Bean Salad with Tuna = 4 mgs
◆ Curried Cream of Wild Rice Soup = 5 mgs
◆ Light Vichyssoise = 5 mgs
◆ Beef and Asparagus in Hot Garlic Sauce = 30 mgs
◆ Oven-Barbecued Pork Tenderloin = 72 mgs
◆ Baked Sea Bass with Shallots and Capers = 58 mgs
◆ Clams and Mussels Marinara = 50 mgs
◆ Spinach Linguine with Walnut Ricotta Sauce = 14 mgs
◆ Pasta with Vodka = 5 mgs
◆ Broccoli with Lemon Mustard Sauce = .3 mg
◆ Twice-Baked Potatoes = 0 mgs
◆ Spiced Peach Soufflé with Fresh Raspberry Sauce = 0 mgs

FEASTS FIT FOR A KING . . . AND FOR YOUR GOOD HEALTH!

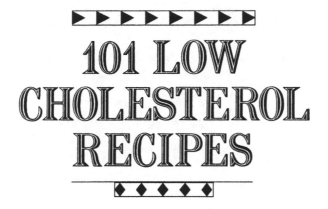

101 LOW CHOLESTEROL RECIPES

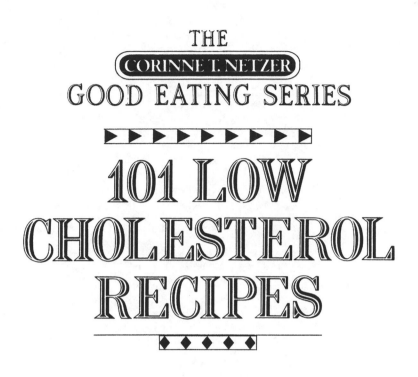

THE CORINNE T. NETZER GOOD EATING SERIES

▶ ▶ ▶ ▶ ▶ ▶ ▶ ▶

101 LOW CHOLESTEROL RECIPES

◆ ◆ ◆ ◆ ◆

Corinne T. Netzer

A Dell Trade Paperback

A DELL TRADE PAPERBACK

Published by
Dell Publishing
a division of
Bantam Doubleday Dell Publishing Group, Inc.
666 Fifth Avenue
New York, New York 10103

Book designed by Rhea Braunstein

Illustrated by Alice Sorensen

Cover photo: Chicken Fricassee, p.83

ISBN: 978-0-440-50417-7

Printed in the United States of America

14691195401

CONTENTS

INTRODUCTION

While almost everyone knows that the U.S. Surgeon General has suggested that we limit our intake of dietary cholesterol to no more than 300 milligrams per day, many people are still confused as to which foods contain this potential menace to good health. Simply put, cholesterol is present only in animal products (meat, poultry, dairy products, and fish).

Certainly we could eliminate all of these items from our menus and thereby kiss dietary cholesterol good-bye, but frankly, why should we? First of all, the cholesterol controversy is far from over. And secondly, I sincerely believe that for most of us it is unnecessary to go to such extremes. My philosophy for producing Good Eating menus is to balance nutrition with variety.

With that in mind, *101 Low Cholesterol Recipes* is not a cholesterol free cookbook, but rather is made up of dishes that keep cholesterol to a minimum without sacrificing good taste.

Each recipe lists the cholesterol count per serving or portion. These figures are derived from information supplied by the United States Department of Agriculture and various food producers and processors.

Here you will find dishes to suit every palate and every occasion, from light to hearty, from simple luncheons to sumptuous dinner parties. And, while the primary focus is on maintaining a low cholesterol count, overall health values have not been ignored.

Enjoy!

C.T.N.

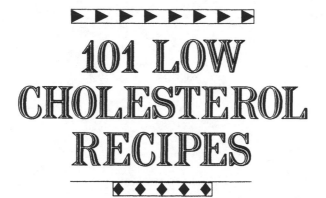

101 LOW
CHOLESTEROL
RECIPES

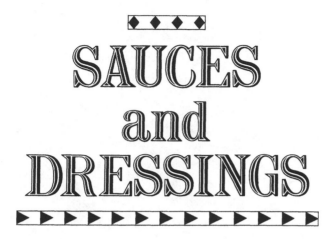

SAUCES and DRESSINGS

The recipes in this section are provided as alternatives to sauces and dressings that are normally high in cholesterol. While it is now possible to find commercial substitutes that are very tasty as well as cholesterol free, many contain exorbitant amounts of fat and sodium.

My recipes have a total fat content that is generally under 30 percent of the calories, and you control the salt shaker.

In the interest of all-around good health, I have opted to formulate recipes with ingredients that contain some dietary cholesterol but are low in fat, rather than utilizing vegetable oils that would result in cholesterol-free dressings and sauces—but with a heavy price: a total fat content of over 90 percent of the calories.

◆ ◆ ◆ ◆ ◆

MOCK SOUR CREAM

▶ ▶

A cup of regular sour cream has 493 calories and an astonishing 102 milligrams of cholesterol! By substituting a cup of store-bought low fat sour cream you can reduce your intake to 280 calories and about 60 milligrams of cholesterol. But, however good store-bought may be (and it *is* good!), I prefer to take the time to make my own. Not only does homemade sour cream give me control over fats and cholesterol, but I am also captain of the ship of salt.

Use wherever you normally would the high-count sour cream.

> 1   *cup low fat (1%) cottage cheese*
> 3   *tablespoons skim milk*
> 1   *tablespoon fresh lemon juice*
>   *Pinch salt, or to taste*

Puree cheese in a blender for 2 minutes. Add milk, lemon juice, and salt, and blend to desired consistency.

MAKES ABOUT 1 CUP
APPROXIMATELY .4 MILLIGRAM CHOLESTEROL
    PER TABLESPOON

◆◆◆◆◆

MOCK MAYONNAISE

▶▶▶▶▶▶▶▶▶▶▶▶▶▶▶▶▶▶▶▶▶▶▶▶▶

The perfect mayonnaise substitute, this spread has the zing of the real thing without the damaging amounts of fat and cholesterol.

Spread it on your sandwiches, mix it in salads, or add additional herbs and spices as I've done in the following recipes, to create a special spread or mayo-type dressing of your own.

> 1   cup low fat plain yogurt
> 1   tablespoon Dijon mustard
> 1/4   teaspoon Worcestershire sauce
> 2   pinches sugar
> 3   tablespoons finely minced onion
>   Pinch salt, or to taste

Combine all ingredients in a small bowl and stir until smoothly mixed. Cover and chill for at least 1 hour to blend flavors. Stir before serving.

MAKES ABOUT 1 CUP
APPROXIMATELY .9 MILLIGRAM CHOLESTEROL
    PER TABLESPOON

◆ ◆ ◆ ◆ ◆

HERBAL MOCK MAYONNAISE
WITH TOFU

▶ ▶

U se this flavored mock mayo to baste grilled poultry or fish, as a spread for crackers, or with just about any kind of salad—crisp greens, tuna, or pasta.

3/4   cup Mock Mayonnaise (page 4)
1/4   cup soft silken tofu
1   tablespoon balsamic vinegar
1   large shallot, minced
2   teaspoons dried parsley
1   teaspoon dried thyme
1/2   teaspoon dried tarragon
   Salt and freshly ground pepper to taste

Combine all ingredients in a blender or food processor. Process for 10 seconds or until smooth. Chill for at least 1 hour before serving to blend flavors.

MAKES ABOUT 1 CUP
APPROXIMATELY .7 MILLIGRAM CHOLESTEROL
PER TABLESPOON

◆◆◆◆◆

GARLIC DIJON
MAYONNAISE-STYLE DRESSING

▶ ▶

For an alternative to crisp greens, toss warm cooked potato cubes, sliced scallions, and crisp-steamed broccoli florets with this dressing for one of the best potato salads ever!

> 1   cup Mock Mayonnaise (see page 4)
> 1   clove garlic, pressed
> 1   tablespoon Dijon mustard, or to taste
> 1   tablespoon white wine vinegar
>   Salt and freshly ground pepper to taste

Combine all ingredients and stir until smoothly mixed. Chill for at least 1 hour before serving to blend flavors.

MAKES ABOUT 1 CUP
APPROXIMATELY .9 MILLIGRAM CHOLESTEROL
    PER TABLESPOON

◆ ◆ ◆ ◆ ◆

LEMON AND BASIL
TOFU DRESSING

▶ ▶

Here's a tangy dressing I like to use for saucing lightly
steamed vegetables such as asparagus, artichokes, string
beans, and cauliflower. Try smearing it in pita pockets,
then fill the pockets with your favorite sandwich stuffers.

  1/2 cup soft silken tofu
   2 tablespoons fresh lemon juice
  1/4 cup minced fresh basil
  1/4 cup low fat buttermilk
      Salt and freshly ground pepper to taste

Combine tofu, lemon juice, basil, and buttermilk in food
processor and blend until mixture is smooth and creamy.
Taste and add salt and pepper, if desired.

MAKES ABOUT 1 CUP
APPROXIMATELY .1 MILLIGRAM CHOLESTEROL PER TABLESPOON

◆ ◆ ◆ ◆ ◆

BUTTERMILK CIDER DRESSING

▶ ▶

A delicious, versatile dressing to use whenever you want to introduce a sweet/tart taste to your salad or platter of crudités.

    ½   cup low fat buttermilk
    2   tablespoons nonfat plain yogurt
    1   tablespoon vegetable oil
    1   tablespoon cider vinegar
    1   tablespoon apple juice
    1   small clove garlic, finely minced
    1   teaspoon grated onion
        Pinch sugar
    ½   teaspoon Dijon mustard
        Salt and freshly ground pepper to taste

Whisk ingredients together and chill for at least 1 hour to blend flavors. You may have to shake or whisk it again just before serving.

MAKES ABOUT 1 CUP
APPROXIMATELY .6 MILLIGRAM CHOLESTEROL
    PER TABLESPOON

◆ ◆ ◆ ◆ ◆

TAHINI YOGURT DRESSING

▶ ▶

U se as a smooth and creamy dressing for fresh green salads or spread on your favorite bread as a gutsy base for turkey or chicken with onion and sprouts.

> ¹/₂ cup nonfat plain yogurt
> 3 tablespoons tahini
> 2 tablespoons fresh lemon juice, or to taste
> 2 tablespoons skim milk
> 1 teaspoon honey
> Salt to taste

Whisk together all ingredients and chill for at least 1 hour to blend flavors.

MAKES ABOUT 1 CUP
APPROXIMATELY .3 MILLIGRAM CHOLESTEROL PER
    TABLESPOON

◆◆◆◆◆

CREAMY BLUE CHEESE DRESSING

▶▶▶▶▶▶▶▶▶▶▶▶▶▶▶▶▶▶▶▶▶▶▶▶

Low in saturated fats and cholesterol, this is one of my favorite reduced-risk dressings. Aside from the usual side-kicks (crudités, salads, sandwiches), try it as a topping for baked small new potatoes.

    ¹/₄   cup evaporated skim milk
    ¹/₄   cup Mock Mayonnaise (page 4)
    ¹/₄   cup Mock Sour Cream (page 3)
    3   tablespoons red wine vinegar
          Pinch dried oregano or marjoram
          Freshly ground pepper to taste
    ³/₄   ounce blue cheese, crumbled

Whisk together all ingredients, except cheese, until creamy and smooth, then stir in cheese. Chill for at least 1 hour to blend flavors.

MAKES ABOUT 1¹/₄ CUPS
APPROXIMATELY 1.0 MILLIGRAM CHOLESTEROL
    PER TABLESPOON

◆ ◆ ◆ ◆ ◆

MEDIUM WHITE SAUCE

▶ ▶

Use this tasty, low cholesterol, low fat sauce whenever the recipe calls for béchamel or a regular white sauce.

> ¹/₄   cup low sodium chicken broth
> 2   tablespoons finely minced shallot (optional)
> 2¹/₂   tablespoons flour
> 1¹/₄   cups low fat (1%) milk
>   Salt and pepper to taste

1. Heat broth in a small saucepan and steam-sauté shallot, if using, over medium-low heat for about 5 minutes or until shallot is very soft. If not using shallot, bring broth to a simmer.

2. Whisk together flour and milk. Pour half of the hot broth into the milk and combine, then pour mixture into saucepan. Cook over medium heat, stirring, until creamy and thickened. Taste, and correct seasonings if necessary.

MAKES ABOUT 1¹/₂ CUPS

APPROXIMATELY 2.0 MILLIGRAMS CHOLESTEROL PER ¹/₄ CUP

◆ ◆ ◆ ◆ ◆

ALL-PURPOSE CURRY SAUCE

▶ ▶

This makes a wonderful dip for raw or crisp-steamed fresh vegetables. I also use it as the dressing for chilled pasta and potato salads and for grilled chicken salad.

> 1 cup Mock Mayonnaise (page 4)
> 1 teaspoon grated ginger root
> 1 tablespoon curry powder, or to taste
> 1/4 teaspoon cayenne, or to taste
> Salt and freshly ground pepper to taste

Combine all ingredients and stir until smooth. Chill for at least 1 hour to blend flavors before serving.

MAKES ABOUT 1 CUP
APPROXIMATELY .9 MILLIGRAM CHOLESTEROL
PER TABLESPOON

◆ ◆ ◆ ◆ ◆

CHEESE SAUCE

▶ ▶

I mitation cheese contains about one-quarter of the cholesterol found in natural cheese. That's good news because there is now a large variety of cheese substitutes available and many good brand choices.

Though zealous cheese purists may shun imitation cheese entirely, when used as an ingredient in a recipe such as this one, it's difficult indeed to tell whether the cheese is natural or imitation—try it.

This sauce is especially good over broccoli, cauliflower, or asparagus, or as a base for macaroni and cheese or any other dish utilizing a cheese sauce.

    2   *tablespoons flour*
    1   *cup evaporated skim milk*
    2   *ounces (¹/₂ cup) imitation low fat cheddar or*
        Swiss cheese, shredded
        Salt to taste
 ¹/₄   *teaspoon hot paprika or dry mustard, or to taste*

1. Whisk together flour and milk in a small nonstick saucepan. Stir over medium heat until mixture is well combined.

2. Reduce heat and stir in cheese, a little at a time. Add salt and paprika or mustard, if desired.

3. Cook, stirring constantly, over very low heat until cheese is melted and ingredients are thoroughly blended.

Serve or use sauce immediately or keep warm over hot water in a double boiler and stir before using.

MAKES ABOUT 1½ CUPS
APPROXIMATELY 2.0 MILLIGRAMS CHOLESTEROL PER ¼ CUP

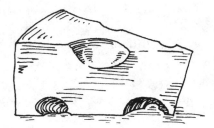

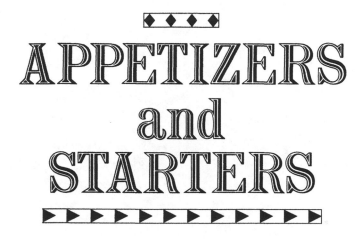

APPETIZERS and STARTERS

◆ ◆ ◆ ◆ ◆

CLAMS IN CUCUMBER CUPS

▶ ▶

You can also use this bold-tasting clam mixture as a topping for halved cherry tomatoes or artichoke hearts, for a spread on melba rounds, or as a dip for bread sticks.

³/₄ *cup drained minced clams, fresh or canned*
1 *teaspoon dry mustard, or to taste*
2 *teaspoons fresh lemon juice*
¹/₄ *cup low fat plain yogurt*
  Salt and freshly ground pepper to taste
1 *teaspoon Worcestershire sauce*
  Pinch cayenne, or to taste
¹/₄ *cup finely minced scallions, white and tender*
  greens
3 *cucumbers, about 9 inches long*
  Paprika
  Parsley sprigs for garnish

1. Combine all ingredients, except scallions, cucumbers, and paprika, in a food processor and process for 3 seconds or until coarsely pureed. Transfer to a mixing bowl and stir in scallions. Refrigerate for at least 1 hour.

2. Cut off ¹/₂ inch from each end of cucumbers. With a fine parer, remove peel and cut each cucumber crosswise into 1-inch-thick slices. Using a melon ball cutter or a small spoon, carefully hollow out the center of each cucumber slice, leaving a thin layer at one end to form a cup.

3. Arrange cucumber cups, open end up, on a serving

---

platter and fill each cup with about 2 teaspoons of clam mixture. Top each with a sprinkle of paprika and serve garnished with parsley sprigs.

MAKES 24 STUFFED CUCUMBER CUPS
APPROXIMATELY 4.0 MILLIGRAMS CHOLESTEROL
    PER CUCUMBER CUP

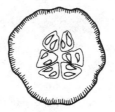

◆ ◆ ◆ ◆ ◆

CURRIED CHICKEN MOUSSE

▶ ▶

Mousse is French for "froth" or "foam" and is used to describe rich, airy dishes that may be sweet or savory, hot or cold. Often fortified with gelatin, their fluffy texture is usually due to the addition of whipped cream or beaten egg whites. This savory mousse has the richness of the traditional dish with only a hint of cholesterol and fat.

Chill the mousse in a 1-quart mold fancy enough to go directly to table.

1	cup dry white wine
1	cup water
1/2	onion, sliced
6	whole peppercorns
1	whole boneless, skinless chicken breast (about 1/2 pound)
1	envelope unflavored gelatin
2	tablespoons cold water
1/3	cup boiling water
1	small onion, quartered
2	teaspoons curry powder, or to taste
2	tablespoons cholesterol-free mayonnaise
3/4	cup nonfat plain yogurt
	Salt and freshly ground pepper to taste
	Wafer-thin lime slices for garnish

1. In a deep skillet or saucepan, combine wine, water, onion slices, and peppercorns. Bring to a boil and simmer for 5 minutes. Add chicken, cover, reduce heat, and simmer

gently for 15 minutes. Remove pot from heat and let chicken cool in the liquid. Keep the lid on the pot. When cooled to room temperature, drain chicken and cut into pieces. Discard cooking liquid.

2. In the bowl of a food processor, sprinkle gelatin over 2 tablespoons water and let stand for 2 minutes. Add boiling water and process quickly with on/off motions until gelatin is dissolved.

3. Add chicken and quartered onion and process until fairly smooth. Add curry powder, mayonnaise, and yogurt and continue processing until mixture is smoothly pureed. Taste and add salt and pepper, if desired.

4. Transfer mixture to a 1-quart mold or serving bowl, cover, and refrigerate for several hours or until set. Serve garnished with lime slices and offer pita triangles and pumpernickel bread.

MAKES ABOUT 3 CUPS
APPROXIMATELY 3.0 MILLIGRAMS CHOLESTEROL
    PER TABLESPOON

◆ ◆ ◆ ◆ ◆

MEATLESS "MEATBALLS"

▶ ▶

$\mathbb{S}$erve these little balls, speared with toothpicks, around a bowl of cool, creamy Herbed Yogurt Dip (page 26), stuff them into a pita pocket with salad greens and Tahini Yogurt Dressing (page 9), or drop them into hot tomato sauce and spoon over pasta. These balls are not only incredibly versatile, but the combination of mushrooms and eggplant gives them a satisfying "meatiness."

1	eggplant (*about 1 pound*)
2	slim zucchini (*about 8 ounces*), *peeled and grated*
2	teaspoons vegetable oil
1/4	pound fresh mushrooms, *wiped clean, coarsely chopped*
1 1/4	cups bread crumbs (*made from 2 to 3 slices day-old Italian bread*)
2	large egg whites
1/2	teaspoon dried marjoram
1/2	teaspoon dried oregano
2	tablespoons minced fresh parsley or 1 tablespoon dried
1/4	cup finely chopped onion, loosely packed
1	medium clove garlic, minced
	Salt and freshly ground pepper to taste

1. Preheat oven to 350°F.

2. Rinse and dry eggplant and roast for 1 hour or until soft when pressed with the back of a spoon. Remove from

oven and let stand until cool enough to handle. Do not turn off oven. When cool, peel eggplant, seed, and coarsely chop pulp.

3. While eggplant roasts, press grated zucchini into a colander, weight with a heavy bowl, and drain for 30 minutes. Squeeze out as much moisture as possible from the drained zucchini and set aside.

4. Heat oil in a nonstick skillet and sauté mushrooms over medium heat until tender.

5. In a large bowl, combine eggplant, zucchini, sautéed mushrooms, and remaining ingredients. Shape into balls about 1¼ inches in diameter and arrange on a broiling rack set into a baking sheet. Cover with foil and bake in the center of oven for 25 minutes. Remove foil and bake for an additional 10 minutes or until balls are golden and crusty.

MAKES 20 TO 24 BALLS
0 MILLIGRAMS CHOLESTEROL PER RECIPE

◆ ◆ ◆ ◆ ◆

SMOKED SALMON–STUFFED EGGS

▶ ▶

$\mathbb{S}$tuffed eggs have always been one of my favorite appetizers. They still are, but now I make them with only the whites, and they're every bit as good as the yolk-filled variety.

This recipe, and the one that follows, are two delicious ways to fill hard-cooked egg whites.

    4   *large hard-cooked egg whites, halved*
    1   *ounce smoked salmon, preferably a nonsalty,*
          nonoily variety, coarsely minced
    1   *tablespoon finely minced red onion*
    2   *teaspoons minced fresh dill weed or 1 teaspoon*
          dried
    2   *teaspoons fresh lemon juice*
          Freshly ground pepper to taste
$^1/_3$ *cup Mock Sour Cream (page 3)*
          Thin lemon slices and parsley sprigs for garnish

1. Place egg whites on a serving dish, cut side up. (To keep the whites from wobbling, cut off a very thin slice from bottoms if it can be done without cutting through the whites.)

2. In a small mixing bowl, combine remaining ingredients and stir until well blended.

3. Spoon stuffing into egg white shells and serve garnished with lemon wedges and parsley, if desired.

MAKES 8 STUFFED EGG HALVES
APPROXIMATELY 1.0 MILLIGRAM CHOLESTEROL PER EGG HALF

◆ ◆ ◆ ◆ ◆

SPINACH-STUFFED EGGS

▶ ▶

　1　teaspoon olive oil
　1　cup chopped fresh spinach leaves, rinsed and
　　　drained
　¹/₃　cup low fat plain yogurt
　1　small clove garlic, finely minced
　1　teaspoon Dijon mustard
　4　large hard-cooked egg whites, halved
　　　Salt and freshly ground pepper to taste

1. Heat oil in a skillet. Add spinach and sauté over medium heat, stirring often, for 5 minutes or until spinach is limp. Drain and discard all excess liquid and transfer spinach to a mixing bowl to cool.

2. Place egg whites on a serving dish, cut side up. (To keep them from wobbling, cut a very thin slice from bottoms if it can be done without cutting through the whites.)

3. Combine yogurt with garlic and mustard and fold into cooled spinach until well blended. Season with salt and pepper, if desired, and spoon spinach mixture into egg halves.

MAKES 8 STUFFED EGG HALVES

APPROXIMATELY .6 MILLIGRAM CHOLESTEROL PER EGG HALF

◆ ◆ ◆ ◆ ◆

LIGHT EGG SALAD

▶ ▶

$\mathbb{S}$erve this yolkless egg salad tucked between two slices of whole-grain bread, cut in thirds for finger sandwiches, or mounded on a plate of chilled greens.

>   5   hard-cooked egg whites, coarsely chopped
>   1/4   cup Mock Mayonnaise (page 4)
>   1/4   cup minced onion
>   1/2   stalk celery, diced
>   1/2   small green bell pepper, finely diced
>   1/2   teaspoon turmeric
>   1/4   teaspoon Dijon mustard, or to taste

Combine all ingredients in a small bowl. Mix just until blended. Cover and refrigerate for 1 hour before serving.

SERVES 4

APPROXIMATELY .9 MILLIGRAM CHOLESTEROL PER SERVING

◆ ◆ ◆ ◆ ◆

HERBED YOGURT DIP

▶ ▶

I nclude this dip as part of a colorful crudités platter. It's also a great accompaniment to curries and spicy meat and poultry dishes. For best results, use fresh herbs.

> 1½ cups low fat plain yogurt
> ¼ cup chopped fresh mint
> 1 tablespoon chopped fresh thyme, oregano, dill, savory, or tarragon (use your favorite blend), or ½ tablespoon dried
> 1 tablespoon fresh lemon juice
> 1 teaspoon honey or sugar
> Salt and freshly ground pepper to taste

Combine all ingredients in a small bowl and chill for 1 hour before serving.

MAKES ABOUT 1¾ CUPS
APPROXIMATELY .8 MILLIGRAM CHOLESTEROL
   PER TABLESPOON

◆ ◆ ◆ ◆ ◆

TOMATO CHEESE CHILI DIP

▶ ▶

S erve with chilled raw vegetables: sliced fresh cucumbers, green, yellow, and red pepper strips, carrot and celery sticks, and zucchini rounds or spears.

  $^1/_2$ cup low fat ricotta cheese
  $^1/_2$ cup low fat (1%) cottage cheese
  1 large ripe tomato, seeded and chopped
  4 scallions, white and tender greens, thinly sliced
  1 small red onion, finely minced
  2 jalapeño peppers, seeded and minced (wear
      rubber gloves), or to taste
  $^1/_2$ tablespoon chili powder, or to taste
  $^1/_4$ cup minced fresh cilantro or parsley
      Salt and freshly ground pepper to taste

Combine all ingredients in a large mixing bowl and stir to blend well. Chill for at least 1 hour before serving.

MAKES ABOUT 2 CUPS
APPROXIMATELY 1.0 MILLIGRAM CHOLESTEROL
  PER TABLESPOON

◆ ◆ ◆ ◆ ◆

CHILLED MUSSELS
WITH SHERRY MUSTARD DIPPING
SAUCE

▶ ▶

This unusual and tangy sauce is the perfect foil for plump, steamed mussels and provides a dish that is equally at home as a member of a cocktail buffet or divided among colorful plates, each dabbed with a little sauce.

> 2   teaspoons olive oil
> 2   large shallots or one small onion, chopped
> 1   cup water
> ¹/₂ cup dry white wine
> 4   dozen mussels, scrubbed and debearded
> 2   teaspoons Dijon mustard
> 1   tablespoon dry sherry
> 1   teaspoon Worcestershire sauce
> 1   teaspoon fresh lemon juice
> ³/₄ cup nonfat plain yogurt
>   Salt and freshly ground pepper to taste
>   Parsley sprigs for garnish

1. Heat oil in a large, deep skillet and sauté shallots or onion over medium-low heat, stirring frequently, until translucent.

2. Add water, wine, and mussels. Raise heat and bring to a boil. Reduce heat slightly, cover, and steam, shaking pan often, for about 6 minutes or until mussels have opened.

3. Using a slotted spoon, remove mussels, discarding any that have not opened. Reserve cooking liquid.

4. When cool enough to handle, remove mussels from shells, place in a bowl or baking dish, barely cover with reserved cooking liquid, and chill. Discard shells.

5. Prepare sauce by combining mustard with sherry, Worcestershire, lemon juice, yogurt, and salt and pepper. Whisk until ingredients are well mixed and transfer to a serving bowl. Chill to blend flavors.

6. Place bowl of sauce in the center of a platter, drain mussels, and arrange around sauce, or divide among six serving plates and garnish with parsley.

SERVES 6

APPROXIMATELY 35.0 MILLIGRAMS CHOLESTEROL PER SERVING

◆ ◆ ◆ ◆ ◆

THREE-BEAN SALAD
WITH TUNA

▶ ▶

This colorful three-bean salad is ideal for hot or cold buffets and makes a good dinner starter. It can also be served as a light warm-weather luncheon salad for four.

Although I've specified canned tuna, if you have any leftover grilled or broiled tuna steaks, swordfish, or salmon, this is an excellent way to use them. Or, if you prefer, omit the fish altogether for a tasty, practically cholesterol free treat.

1/2 *pound green beans, trimmed, crisp-steamed, and cooled*
1/2 *pound wax (yellow) beans, trimmed, crisp-steamed, and cooled*
1 *cup black beans, cooked or canned, rinsed, and drained*
1 *small red onion, chopped*
1 *stalk celery, diced*
1/2 *red bell pepper, seeded and diced*
3 *ounces water-packed light tuna, drained and flaked*
1/3 *cup white wine vinegar or cider vinegar*
1/2 *cup low sodium chicken broth*
2 *tablespoons olive oil*
1 *teaspoon dry mustard*
2 *cloves garlic, pressed*
1 *tablespoon minced fresh parsley or basil*

Salt and freshly ground pepper to taste
Lettuce leaves and tomato wedges

1. Cut green and wax beans into 1-inch lengths and place in a large mixing bowl. Add black beans, onion, celery, bell pepper, and tuna. Toss lightly to combine.

2. In a small bowl or jar with a tight-fitting lid, combine vinegar, broth, oil, mustard, garlic, and parsley or basil. Stir or shake well to blend. Taste and add salt and pepper, if desired.

3. Pour dressing over bean mixture and toss lightly. Refrigerate for at least 2 hours to blend flavors. Toss again before serving.

4. Cover a serving platter or individual dishes with lettuce leaves, top with chilled salad, surround with tomato wedges, and serve.

SERVES 8

APPROXIMATELY 4.0 MILLIGRAMS CHOLESTEROL PER SERVING

◆ ◆ ◆ ◆ ◆

CELERIAC REMOULADE

▶ ▶

Celeriac (also known as celery root) is the ugly duckling of vegetables—coarse-skinned, brown, knobby. But when its exterior is peeled away and the delicate flesh is combined with a creamy mustard-laced sauce, the result is a dish beautiful and elegant enough to grace any table.

My version of this classic French appetizer is very low in fat and cholesterol, but you'd never know it.

> 1   *small celeriac (about 3/4 pound)*
> 1   *tablespoon lemon juice*
> 1   *cup Mock Mayonnaise (page 4)*
> 1   *tablespoon Dijon mustard, or to taste*
> 2   *teaspoons capers, rinsed and drained*

1. Cut off brown, knobby peel of celeriac and shred the flesh (a food processor fitted with a fine shredding disk works well). Transfer celeriac to a mixing bowl and toss quickly with lemon juice to keep it from discoloring.

2. Combine remaining ingredients. Add to celeriac and toss until well coated. Refrigerate for several hours to blend flavors before serving.

SERVES 6

APPROXIMATELY 2.0 MILLIGRAMS CHOLESTEROL PER SERVING

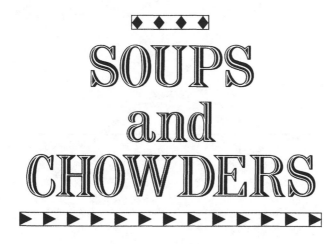

SOUPS and CHOWDERS

♦ ♦ ♦ ♦ ♦

CREAM OF KALE AND POTATO SOUP

▶ ▶

One of the most pleasant memories of my childhood has to do with kale and Agnes Johnson, my friend from Alabama. Dinner with Agnes's family was my introduction to the wonders of Deep South–style home cooking. Agnes's mother was a robust woman with a loud, easy laugh. Her cooking was generous: in amounts served, color, texture, and eye appeal. It may have lacked finesse, but great balls of fire, what taste!

My favorite was a dish consisting of pan-fried cornmeal topped with an exotic-looking blue-tinged, deep-green frilly vegetable. Later I was to discover this green stuff was kale.

My love affair with this unusual member of the cabbage family has continued, and I use kale in a host of dishes, frequently substituting it for spinach. Packing a Popeye-strong punch, kale provides substantial amounts of vitamins A and C, folic acid, calcium, and iron. When grouped with the rest of the ingredients for my soup, it produces one of the most truly sublime dishes this side of Mrs. Johnson's.

1   *large onion, diced*
2   *cloves garlic, minced*
1   *tablespoon olive oil*
4   *small potatoes, peeled and diced*
2   *cups water*
2   *cups evaporated skim milk*

$^3/_4$ *pound kale, rinsed, trimmed, and finely shredded*
    Salt and freshly ground pepper to taste

1. In a large saucepan, sauté onion and garlic in oil over medium-low heat until soft.
2. Add potatoes and water. Cover and cook over low heat for 15 to 20 minutes or until potatoes are tender. Stir in milk and bring to a simmer, but do not boil.
3. Puree potato-milk mixture in blender or food processor until smooth. Return to saucepan.
4. Add kale and season with salt and pepper, if desired. Cover and cook over very low heat for 15 minutes or until kale is tender.

SERVES 4

APPROXIMATELY 3.0 MILLIGRAMS CHOLESTEROL PER SERVING

◆ ◆ ◆ ◆

AVGOLEMONO
WITH CHICKEN AND RICE

▶ ▶

A great favorite in Greece and the Mideast, this delicious soup is traditionally thickened with egg yolks. I have found that cornstarch does the job just as well and makes it possible for the cholesterol-conscious to enjoy this luscious lemony soup without guilt.

If you prefer, a tiny pasta (orzo or pastina) or barley can be substituted for the rice.

    4   cups low sodium chicken broth
  1¹/₂ cups water
   ¹/₂ boneless, skinless chicken breast (about 5 ounces),
        diced
   ¹/₂ cup uncooked rice
    1   teaspoon dried parsley
    3   tablespoons fresh lemon juice, or to taste
        Salt and freshly ground pepper to taste
    2   tablespoons cornstarch
        Chopped fresh chives or minced scallions for
        garnish

1. Combine broth and 1 cup water in a large kettle and bring to a boil. Reduce heat, add chicken, rice, parsley, lemon juice, and salt and pepper to taste. Cover and simmer gently for 20 minutes.

2. Dissolve cornstarch in remaining ¹/₂ cup water and

add to soup. Cook over medium heat, stirring often, for 5 minutes.

3. Transfer soup to a tureen or individual bowls, sprinkle with chives or scallions, and serve.

SERVES 4
APPROXIMATELY 25.0 MILLIGRAMS CHOLESTEROL PER SERVING

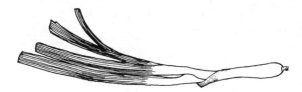

◆ ◆ ◆ ◆

MUSSEL CHOWDER

▶ ▶

Although mussels have long been prized throughout Europe as one of the greatest mollusks ever to hit a kettle for steaming, they have not yet completely caught the fancy of American foodies. And so much the loss! Because mussels are one of the finest choices for heart-healthy feasting (1 ounce of steamed mussel meat contains only 1 gram of fat, a trace of saturated fat, 16 milligrams of cholesterol, and 49 calories).

Cleaning the mussels is the only drawback to the preparation of any mussel dish. While it's true that farmed mussels sometimes come to the market fairly well scrubbed and debearded, frequently this tedious procedure is left up to us. However, once you have gotten past this joyless task, the rest of the work goes quickly and the results are compellingly rewarding.

This soothing, satisfying chowder has an aroma and flavor that is sheer heaven. Serve with toasted French bread rounds rubbed with garlic.

1¹/₂   cups dry white wine
¹/₂   cup water
2   dozen mussels, scrubbed and debearded
1   tablespoon oil, preferably olive
1   small onion, chopped
1   stalk celery, diced
¹/₄   cup chopped green bell pepper
¹/₄   cup chopped red bell pepper
¹/₂   cup diced carrots

1 28-ounce can no-salt-added plum tomatoes in
   juice, chopped, or 3 large, ripe tomatoes, peeled
   and chopped, juice reserved
2 medium round potatoes, peeled and cubed
1 bay leaf
   Pinch dried tarragon
1 cup fish stock or clam broth
   Salt and freshly ground pepper to taste

1. Combine 1 cup wine and water in a large stockpot or kettle and bring to a boil. Reduce heat slightly, add mussels, cover, and steam over medium heat, shaking pot occasionally, for about 6 minutes or until mussels have opened.

2. Using a slotted spoon, transfer mussels to a bowl, discarding any that have not opened. Strain cooking liquid through a fine sieve lined with cheesecloth, and reserve. Remove mussels from shells, discard shells, and wipe out kettle.

3. Heat oil in kettle, add onion, celery, bell peppers, and carrots and sauté over medium heat until onion is translucent and vegetables begin to soften.

4. Raise heat to medium-high, add tomatoes with juice, strained cooking liquid, remaining ½ cup wine, potatoes, bay leaf, tarragon, and stock or broth. Bring to a boil, cover, lower heat, and simmer for 20 minutes. Add mussels and simmer for an additional 10 minutes or until potatoes are cooked through. Taste and add salt and pepper, if desired.

SERVES 4
APPROXIMATELY 34.0 MILLIGRAMS CHOLESTEROL PER SERVING

♦ ♦ ♦ ♦ ♦

CURRIED CREAM OF WILD RICE SOUP

▶ ▶

This unusual soup is so satisfying, you can easily build an entire meal around it.

>   1   *tablespoon olive oil*
>   3   *cloves garlic, minced*
>   ¹/₂   *cup finely diced onion*
>   ¹/₂   *cup diced celery*
>   2   *tablespoons flour*
>   4   *cups water or vegetable broth, approximately*
>   1   *tablespoon curry powder, or to taste*
>   ¹/₂   *teaspoon turmeric*
>   ¹/₈   *teaspoon ground coriander (optional)*
>   ³/₄   *cup nonfat dry milk*
>   ¹/₂   *cup diced carrots*
>   1¹/₂   *cups cooked wild rice*
>   *Salt and freshly ground pepper to taste*

1. Heat oil in large nonstick kettle or stockpot over low heat and sauté garlic, onion, and celery, stirring frequently, until vegetables are wilted.

2. Sprinkle vegetables with flour and stir until flour dissolves. Raise heat to medium, pour in ¹/₄ cup water or broth, and cook, stirring, for about 2 minutes. Add curry powder, turmeric, and coriander.

3. Add remaining liquid and sprinkle with nonfat dry milk, stirring to dissolve. Add carrots and rice, cover, and

simmer gently for about 15 minutes or until carrots are tender. Add more liquid, ¼ cup at a time, if needed. Taste and add salt and pepper, if desired.

SERVES 4

APPROXIMATELY 5.0 MILLIGRAMS CHOLESTEROL PER SERVING

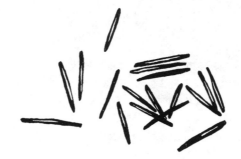

◆ ◆ ◆ ◆ ◆

BORSCHT

▶ ▶

There are about as many recipes for borscht as there are Russian cooks, and almost as many ways to serve it. I like my borscht served hot with the vegetables chunky, but if you prefer, the soup can be strained or pureed and served chilled.

However you serve this tasty soup, just about everyone agrees it goes well with sour cream (fear not, I use Mock Sour Cream) and huge slices of pumpernickel or Russian black bread.

    2   medium beets, peeled and quartered
    1   carrot, cut into 2-inch lengths
    1   medium onion, quartered
    1   cup finely shredded cabbage
   4½   cups water
    1   cup low sodium tomato sauce
    2   tablespoons red wine vinegar
    1   teaspoon sugar (optional)
         Salt and freshly ground pepper to taste
    4   tablespoons Mock Sour Cream (page 3)

1. Grate beets, carrot, and onion, using a hand grater or the fine grater of a food processor.

2. Transfer grated vegetables to a large kettle or stockpot and add cabbage and water. Bring to a boil, cover, reduce heat to low, and simmer gently for 45 minutes.

3. Add tomato sauce, vinegar, sugar if desired, and salt

and pepper to taste. Stir, cover, and cook over low heat for an additional 30 minutes.

4. Serve hot or chilled in individual bowls, each topped with a tablespoon of Mock Sour Cream.

SERVES 4

APPROXIMATELY .4 MILLIGRAM CHOLESTEROL PER SERVING

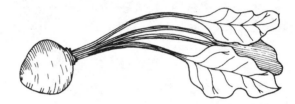

◆ ◆ ◆ ◆ ◆

CANTONESE SOUR SOUP
WITH SPINACH

▶ ▶

R uby Foo's was The Place to Go in Manhattan for Chinese food until its demise in the late '70s. Many New Yorkers embraced the gooey meals Ruby's dished up as authentic Cantonese cuisine when nothing could have been further from the truth. In reality, Cantonese cuisine is marked by its delicate sauces and the use of the freshest ingredients available.

I have long since discovered the infinite pleasures of good Cantonese cooking from the remarkable restaurants that dot New York's Chinatown. My sour soup pays humble homage to the epicurean miracles of Chinese-style cooking.

4   *cups low sodium chicken broth*
¹/₄   *pound lean pork tenderloin, trimmed of all visible*
      fat and cut into thin strips (this task is easier if
      the meat is partially frozen)
¹/₂   *cup canned, drained, and sliced bamboo shoots*
2   *dried Chinese mushrooms*, soaked in warm*
      water for 30 minutes, drained, stemmed, and
      sliced
¹/₄   *cup canned, drained, and sliced water chestnuts*
8   *ounces tofu, diced*
1   *tablespoon sake (rice wine) or dry sherry*
1   *tablespoon low sodium soy sauce*
1   *tablespoon red wine vinegar*

Freshly ground pepper to taste
2   *tablespoons cornstarch*
¹/₄ *cup cold water*
¹/₂ *pound fresh spinach, rinsed, drained, and cut
into long strips
Salt to taste*
1   *scallion, white and tender greens, thinly sliced*

1. Heat broth in a large kettle or stockpot over medium flame. When it boils, add pork, bamboo shoots, mushrooms, and water chestnuts. Cover, reduce heat, and simmer gently for 15 minutes.

2. Add tofu, sake, soy sauce, vinegar, and several grindings of black pepper. Return liquid to a simmer.

3. Dissolve cornstarch in cold water and stir into soup. Simmer, stirring frequently, until soup thickens.

4. Stir in spinach and swirl just until wilted. Taste and add salt, if desired. Ladle into bowls and sprinkle with sliced scallion. Serve very hot.

SERVES 4

APPROXIMATELY 23.0 MILLIGRAMS CHOLESTEROL PER SERVING

* Available at Oriental and specialty food markets

◆ ◆ ◆ ◆ ◆

CREAMY CORN AND LIMA SOUP
(Adapted from Josephine DiDonato)

▶ ▶

How many of us remember our first meeting with that pale green, voluptuous, kidney-curved bean called The Lima? Mine occurred in grammar school where we examined the lima's germination, which was taking place inelegantly between a blotter and the side of a glass. We dutifully watered it and watched it grow, right before our awe-filled eyes.

At that time in my life examining the lima was a far more rewarding experience than eating it. Suffering with succotash? You bet I suffered! That is, until my dear friend Josephine illuminated the virtues of this venerable combination of corn with baby lima beans in her zesty and delightful Creamy Corn and Lima Soup, which I pass along to you.

2   teaspoons unsalted margarine
1   large leek, white and 1 inch of tender greens,
    well rinsed and chopped
3   cups low sodium chicken broth
1   cup water
2   cups baby lima beans, fresh, or frozen and thawed
1   cup corn kernels, fresh, or frozen and thawed
1   small mild green chili pepper, seeded and
    chopped
1/4   teaspoon dried thyme
    Salt and freshly ground pepper to taste

$^{1}/_{2}$ cup low fat buttermilk
     Pinch nutmeg
  2   tablespoons chopped fresh chives

1. Heat margarine in a large soup pot. Add leek and cook over medium heat, stirring frequently, until well wilted.

2. Add 2 cups broth, the water, lima beans, corn, chili pepper, thyme, and salt and pepper to taste, and bring mixture to a boil. Reduce heat and simmer gently, uncovered, for about 30 minutes or until beans and leeks are very tender. Check pot occasionally and add broth as liquid evaporates until all broth is used.

3. Reduce heat to very low and stir in buttermilk and nutmeg. Mixture should not boil after the buttermilk is added. Remove pot from heat if necessary. When soup is heated through, sprinkle with chives and serve immediately.

SERVES 4

APPROXIMATELY 5.0 MILLIGRAMS CHOLESTEROL PER SERVING

◆ ◆ ◆ ◆ ◆

HEARTY CABBAGE SOUP
WITH VEGETABLES AND BEEF

▶ ▶

This substantial and earthy soup is perfect fare for the coldest days of winter. Served with a simple green salad, the combination of ingredients makes a satisfying meal. If you have any left over, store it in the refrigerator or freezer—it's even better reheated.

2	teaspoons vegetable oil
³/₄	pound boneless lean beef, trimmed of all visible fat and cut in ³/₄-inch cubes
2	medium onions, diced
2	stalks celery, diced
3	large cloves garlic, minced
4¹/₂	cups water
4	cups low sodium beef or chicken broth
³/₄	cup dry red wine
2	tablespoons red wine vinegar
1	28-ounce can no-salt-added plum tomatoes with juice, chopped
1	bay leaf
2	tablespoons minced fresh parsley or 1 tablespoon dried
1	teaspoon dried oregano
1	teaspoon dried thyme
1	teaspoon dried basil
	Salt and freshly ground pepper to taste
2	medium parsnips, peeled and diced

4 medium potatoes, peeled and diced
1 head green cabbage (about 1¼ pounds),
   quartered, cored, and coarsely shredded

1. Heat oil in a large nonstick skillet. Add beef and cook over medium-high heat, stirring often, for about 5 minutes or until browned. Using a slotted spoon, transfer beef to a large stockpot or kettle.

2. Add onions, celery, and garlic to skillet. Cook over medium heat, stirring often, for 3 minutes or until onion is translucent. Transfer contents of skillet to pot containing the beef.

3. Add water, broth, wine, vinegar, tomatoes, bay leaf, parsley, oregano, thyme, basil, and salt and pepper to beef in pot. Stir to combine ingredients, and bring to a boil. Reduce heat to very low, cover, and simmer gently for 45 minutes.

4. Add parsnips and potatoes to pot. Cover, and simmer for an additional 20 minutes.

5. Stir cabbage into pot, adding additional water if mixture is very thick. Cover and simmer gently for 15 minutes. Taste and adjust seasonings, if necessary.

SERVES 8

APPROXIMATELY 25.0 MILLIGRAMS CHOLESTEROL PER SERVING

◆ ◆ ◆ ◆ ◆

LIGHT VICHYSSOISE

▶ ▶

Vichyssoise, that wonderful French-inspired blend of rich broth, butter, and heavy cream (with some leeks and potatoes thrown in), has long been one of my favorite chilled soups. So years ago when I started to watch my dietary cholesterol and fat intake and cook accordingly, concocting a low cholesterol, low fat replica that would retain the taste and flavor of a classic vichyssoise became a challenge. This Light Vichyssoise is a very able substitute.

1   *tablespoon unsalted margarine*
2   *medium leeks, white bulbs only, well rinsed and*
    coarsely chopped
1   *small onion, chopped*
1   *clove garlic, chopped*
1   *cup water*
2   *cups low sodium chicken broth*
2   *medium potatoes, peeled and diced*
1   *cup evaporated skim milk*
    Salt and freshly ground pepper to taste
2   *tablespoons minced scallions or chopped fresh*
    chives for garnish

1. Heat margarine in a soup pot. Add leeks, onion, and garlic and cook, stirring often, over medium-low heat for 5 minutes or until leeks are softened but not browned.

2. Stir in water and broth and add potatoes. Cover, reduce heat to low, and simmer for about 30 minutes or until potatoes are very tender. Remove from heat and cool slightly.

---

3. Transfer contents of pot to a food processor and puree until smooth, then return to pot.

4. Stir milk into soup and cook over very low heat until well blended and heated through. Do not boil. Remove from heat and cool to room temperature.

5. Cover and refrigerate for at least 4 hours. Stir well and transfer to chilled individual bowls or a tureen, and serve garnished with scallions or chives.

SERVES 4

APPROXIMATELY 5.0 MILLIGRAMS CHOLESTEROL PER SERVING

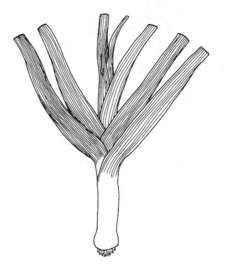

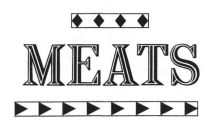

MEATS

◆ ◆ ◆ ◆ ◆

BEEF SUKIYAKI STYLE

▶ ▶

Sukiyaki may be Japan's answer to America's chili, India's curry, or Italy's pasta—dishes that seem to appeal to just about everybody. In fact, sukiyaki is known as the "friendship dish" by the Japanese because it is a favorite of foreigners. And why not? Appealing to behold, aromatic, tasty, and nutritionally sound, this one-dish meal is an all-around winner.

Sukiyaki consists of bite-size pieces of meat, vegetables, tofu, and occasionally noodles, flavored with soy, spices, and sake, the fragrant Japanese rice wine. It is essential that the beef be sliced razor-thin, so be sure the meat is partially frozen for easy slicing—or, better yet, ask a sympathetic butcher to perform this operation for you.

Sukiyaki is a simple yet showy dish that is best shown off when prepared at the table in an electric wok or skillet. Have all the ingredients ready before you cook, and serve with Oriental noodles (soba, udon, or cellophane*) or with plain rice.

1	tablespoon vegetable oil
3/4	pound very lean beef eye round, trimmed of all visible fat and very thinly sliced
2	tablespoons sugar
1/2	cup low sodium beef broth
1/4	cup mirin*
8	ounces firm tofu, thinly sliced
8	fresh shiitake mushrooms*, wiped clean, sliced

1 medium carrot, shaved lengthwise into ribbons
  (use a vegetable parer)
2 small leeks, white and tender greens, well rinsed
  and sliced diagonally into 1-inch lengths
½ package rice sticks*
1 pound young Swiss chard, bok choy, or napa
  cabbage, tough stems trimmed, well rinsed, large
  leaves cut in half lengthwise

1. Heat oil in wok or large nonstick skillet, tilting it to distribute a thin, even film. Add beef and sauté quickly until beef just begins to lose its raw look, pushing it around with chopsticks or a wooden spoon (this may have to be done in two or three steps). Remove beef and set aside.

2. Mix together sugar, broth, and mirin and add to wok. Add tofu and mushrooms and stir. Cook for 3 minutes. Add carrot, leeks, and rice sticks and cook for another 2 minutes. Add Swiss chard and swirl with chopsticks.

3. Return beef to sauce, heat through, and serve.

SERVES 4
APPROXIMATELY 57.0 MILLIGRAMS CHOLESTEROL
    PER SERVING

* Available at health food or specialty stores, and Oriental markets.

◆ ◆ ◆ ◆ ◆

MOROCCAN BEEF AND VEGETABLES GRILLED ON SKEWERS

▶ ▶

I am a big fan of any kind of cooking that will produce Good Eating in short order. So it is little wonder that high on my list are foods cooked on skewers. Whether called *brochette, shish kebab, shashlik, satay,* or *yakatori,* the technique is basically the same.

Generally, fish, chicken, or meat is cut into bite-size pieces, marinated, and skewered, often with vegetables and/or fruits. The skewered foods are then placed on the grill or under the broiler (about 5 inches from the source of heat), and turned and basted as they cook.

Serve this Moroccan-inspired dish with such kindred souls as chick-pea salad with fresh greens and my Tahini Yogurt Dressing (page 9).

¹/₂	cup seedless raisins, chopped
1	cup dry red wine
1	cup low sodium beef broth
³/₄	cup finely chopped onion
1	teaspoon ground ginger
1	teaspoon turmeric
	Salt and freshly ground pepper to taste
³/₄	pound lean beef top round, trimmed of all visible fat and cubed
1¹/₄	pounds turnips, peeled and cubed
2	slender zucchini (about 4 ounces each), ends trimmed, cut into ¹/₂-inch slices

> 12 cherry tomatoes
> 12 small boiling onions, peeled

1. Combine raisins, wine, broth, and chopped onion in a small saucepan. Bring to a boil, stirring, then remove from heat and let cool. Stir in ginger, turmeric, and salt and pepper. Transfer mixture to a baking dish, and add beef cubes. Toss to coat, cover, and marinate in refrigerator for at least 1 hour.

2. Prepare grill or preheat broiler.

3. Reserving marinade, remove beef and thread onto skewers, alternating beef cubes with turnips, zucchini, tomatoes, and whole small onions. Grill or broil meat and vegetable skewers until beef is cooked to desired degree of doneness, turning skewers and basting occasionally with marinade. Serve on a large platter or remove meat and vegetables from skewers and divide among six plates.

SERVES 6

APPROXIMATELY 23.0 MILLIGRAMS CHOLESTEROL PER SERVING

◆ ◆ ◆ ◆ ◆

SAVORY ROLLED STEAK

▶ ▶

This dish is a good choice for a dinner party; it's easy to prepare but doesn't look it, and it goes well with just about anything. I like to serve it with pureed chestnuts.

Don't cut the marination time short—flank steak, a long, thin, fibrous, and lean cut of beef, benefits greatly from marinating, and the longer it sits the more tender the meat will be.

> 2   teaspoons vegetable oil
> 1   small onion, minced
> 1/4 cup finely diced carrot
> 1/4 cup chopped fresh parsley
> 2   pounds flank steak, in one piece, trimmed of all
>   visible fat
>   Salt and freshly ground pepper to taste
> 1   tablespoon grated Romano cheese
> 1/2 cup dry red wine
> 2   tablespoons red wine vinegar
> 1   large clove garlic, pressed

1. Heat oil in a medium nonstick skillet. Add onion and carrot and cook over medium heat, stirring often, for 3 minutes. Stir in parsley and remove skillet from heat.

2. Sprinkle one side of steak with salt and pepper to taste, spread with onion-parsley mixture nearly to edge of meat, and sprinkle with grated cheese. Beginning at narrow end, roll up steak and secure with string, skewers, or toothpicks.

---

3. Combine wine, vinegar, and garlic in a shallow baking dish. Add rolled beef, turning to coat all sides with marinade, cover and refrigerate for at least 4 hours, turning meat occasionally.

4. Preheat oven to 375°F.

5. Place rolled steak in a shallow roasting pan and roast in oven, uncovered, for about 45 minutes or until tender, basting occasionally with any reserved marinade and turning meat two or three times during cooking. Remove from oven, allow meat to stand for 5 minutes, then remove string, skewers, or toothpicks. Cut roast crosswise into thin slices and serve.

SERVES 8

APPROXIMATELY 45.0 MILLIGRAMS CHOLESTEROL PER SERVING

◆ ◆ ◆ ◆ ◆

BEEF AND ASPARAGUS
IN HOT GARLIC SAUCE

▶ ▶

This classic Chinese stir-fry dish cooks in no time at all.
Serve it with brown rice and fortune cookies.

1	pound fresh asparagus
1	teaspoon peanut oil
1	teaspoon sesame oil
1/2	pound beef top round, trimmed of all visible fat and sliced into thin strips (partially freeze meat to make slicing easier)
2	large cloves garlic, chopped
2	dried Chinese hot red pepper pods, uncracked, or pinch flakes
3/4	cup low sodium beef broth
1	teaspoon sugar (optional)
1	tablespoon low sodium soy sauce
1	teaspoon red wine vinegar
4	scallions, white and tender greens, thinly sliced

1. Rinse asparagus and snap off tough stems. If asparagus stalks are thick, cut them in half lengthwise, then cut diagonally into 1 1/2-inch lengths crosswise. If stalks are thin, just cut them crosswise.

2. Heat oils in a nonstick wok or deep skillet over medium-high heat. Add asparagus and stir-fry for 2 minutes. Remove skillet from heat and remove asparagus.

3. Return skillet to heat. Add beef, garlic, and hot pepper and cook, stirring, over high heat for 30 seconds.

---

4. Add broth, sugar if desired, and soy sauce. When mixture starts to boil, return asparagus to pan, stir in vinegar and scallions, and cook for 2 minutes. Remove pepper pods before serving.

SERVES 4

APPROXIMATELY 30.0 MILLIGRAMS CHOLESTEROL PER SERVING

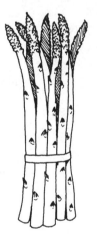

◆◆◆◆◆

MOUSSAKA
WITH POTATO CRUST

▶ ▶

A gift from the Greeks, moussaka is popular throughout most of the Near East. Moussaka basically consists of layers of sliced eggplant and ground lamb or beef, but the variations are virtually limitless. The dish is sometimes covered with a béchamel sauce that has been enriched with eggs and/or cheese or with the addition of onions, artichokes, tomatoes, or potatoes.

I have streamlined the recipe for a Good-Eating life-style by increasing the proportion of eggplant to meat and substituting potatoes for the béchamel topping, thus making it a nutritionally acceptable taste-pleaser.

2   medium eggplants (about 1¹/₄ pounds each)
1   tablespoon olive oil
    Vegetable oil cooking spray
2   large onions, chopped
2   large cloves garlic, chopped
1   pound lean lamb, trimmed of all visible fat and
    ground (have the butcher do it)
2   cups canned no-salt-added tomatoes with puree,
    chopped
¹/₂ cup full-bodied red wine
    Pinch ground allspice
    Pinch ground cinnamon
¹/₂ teaspoon dried oregano
3   tablespoons chopped fresh parsley or 1¹/₂
    tablespoons dried

3   *medium potatoes, peeled and halved*
¹/₄ *cup skim milk*
    Salt and freshly ground pepper to taste

1. Rinse eggplant and cut into ¹/₄-inch-thick slices. Lay slices in a colander, sprinkle lightly with salt if desired, cover the slices with a heavy plate or bowl, and drain for 30 minutes.

2. Preheat broiler.

3. Rinse eggplant well, pat dry, and broil about 5 inches from heat source, turning slices once, until golden on both sides. Remove from oven and set aside. Reset oven to 350°F.

4. Heat oil in a large skillet coated with cooking spray. Add onions and cook over medium-low heat, stirring occasionally, until soft.

5. Add garlic and, if additional moisture is needed, a tablespoon or two of the wine, and continue to cook until onions are lightly golden.

6. Add lamb to onions, raise heat to medium, and brown lamb, breaking up any clumps of meat with a wooden spoon. When lamb is lightly browned, drain off all accumulated fat from the skillet and add tomatoes, wine, allspice, cinnamon, and oregano. Cook, stirring occasionally, until liquid is reduced and mixture is slightly thickened. Stir in parsley.

7. While mixture cooks, boil potatoes for about 20 minutes or until tender. Drain and mash with the skim milk and salt and pepper to taste.

8. Coat a 9- by 13-inch baking pan lightly with cooking spray and arrange a layer of eggplant on the bottom. Follow with some of the lamb mixture, and repeat procedure until ingredients are all layered into the pan, ending with eggplant slices. Top the casserole with the mashed potatoes, smoothing with a spatula. Cover with foil and bake for 30 minutes,

then remove foil and bake for an additional 15 minutes or until top is crusty.

SERVES 6
APPROXIMATELY 45.0 MILLIGRAMS CHOLESTEROL PER SERVING

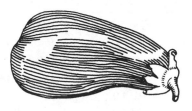

◆ ◆ ◆ ◆ ◆

LAMB AND VEGETABLE BURGERS

▶ ▷

If you love burgers but have given them up for the obvious reasons, try these—meat is not their sole ingredient, yet the taste holds up. If you prefer, use lean ground beef in place of the lamb (the cholesterol content is very similar). For vegetarians and those on strict cholesterol free diets, a cup of mashed chick-peas may be substituted for the lamb.

Serve on whole wheat buns with all your favorite trimmings: tomato, lettuce, onions, etc. Or stuff into pita pockets with shredded lettuce and a tablespoon of my Tahini Yogurt Dressing (page 9).

6	*ounces lean ground lamb*
1	*stalk celery, finely diced*
1	*small carrot, shredded or grated*
1	*small onion, finely minced*
1	*clove garlic, minced*
1	*teaspoon ground ginger*
1	*teaspoon dried parsley*
1/4	*cup whole wheat flour*
1	*cup dry bread crumbs*
1	*egg white*
	Salt and freshly ground pepper to taste
1	*tablespoon peanut oil*
	Vegetable oil cooking spray

1. In a large mixing bowl, combine lamb with all remaining ingredients, except oil and cooking spray, and mix until thoroughly blended.

---

66 ◆ *101 Low Cholesterol Recipes/Corinne T. Netzer*

2. Divide into 4 equal portions and shape into patties, packing mixture firmly.

3. Heat oil in a nonstick skillet coated with cooking spray. Add patties and cook until golden brown on both sides.

SERVES 4

APPROXIMATELY 29.0 MILLIGRAMS CHOLESTEROL PER SERVING

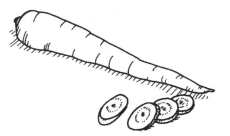

◆◆◆◆◆

OVEN-BARBECUED
PORK TENDERLOIN

▶▶▶▶▶▶▶▶▶▶▶▶▶▶▶▶▶▶▶▶▶▶▶▶▶

Thanks to improved breeding and feeding methods, to-day's pork is leaner (about a third fewer calories) and higher in protein than it was just ten years ago. In addition, the fat in pork is somewhat less saturated than beef's, its cholesterol content is lower than veal's, and it is an excellent source of B vitamins (particularly thiamine), zinc, and iron.

Pork tenderloin, a very lean cut that can easily dry out if overcooked, is often marinated to add moisture and tenderness as well as flavor. The marinade in this dish produces the delicious barbecue taste usually associated with high fat spareribs.

> *Vegetable oil cooking spray*
> 1 *teaspoon vegetable oil*
> 1½ *tablespoons finely minced or grated onion*
> 2 *medium cloves garlic, finely minced, or to taste*
> 1 *tablespoon tomato paste (preferably sun-dried)*
> ½ *tablespoon sugar or honey*
> 1 *tablespoon light brown sugar*
> 1 *teaspoon Worcestershire sauce*
> 1½ *tablespoons red wine vinegar*
> ½ *cup orange juice*
> ¼ *teaspoon cayenne, or to taste*
> 1 *pound pork tenderloin, trimmed of all visible fat*

---

1. Heat a skillet coated with cooking spray and oil and sauté onion and garlic over medium heat until softened but not brown. Stir in tomato paste and cook for 1 minute. Add remaining ingredients, except pork, and simmer, stirring occasionally, for about 10 minutes. Marinade can be refrigerated overnight.

2. Lay tenderloin into a shallow dish and dress with marinade, turning the pork to coat all sides. Cover and refrigerate for at least 2 hours.

3. Preheat oven to 350°F.

4. Transfer tenderloin to a shallow pan and roast, basting occasionally with marinade, for about 50 minutes or until pork is just cooked through but not dry.

SERVES 4

APPROXIMATELY 72.0 MILLIGRAMS CHOLESTEROL PER SERVING

◆ ◆ ◆ ◆

PORK AND WINTER SQUASH

▶ ▶

Winter squash varieties include acorn, buttercup, pumpkin, hubbard, and butternut. All squashes are a good source of fiber, and a cup of baked squash provides almost one and a half times the vitamin A (in the form of beta carotene) needed daily, plus an ample amount of potassium.

Butternut is one of the most popular of the winter squashes. Pear-shaped, with a sweet, orange flesh, it can weigh from 2 to 5 pounds or more, and can be baked, steamed, or simmered—as it is here, with lean pork in a tasty sauce.

Steamed greens, such as spinach, Swiss chard, or collards, make a colorful addition.

> 2 tablespoons medium-dry sherry
> 1 tablespoon low sodium soy sauce
> 1 tablespoon fresh lemon juice
> ³/₄ pound lean pork tenderloin, trimmed of all visible fat and sliced ¹/₂ inch thick, slices cut in half crosswise
> Vegetable oil cooking spray
> 3 teaspoons peanut oil
> 1¹/₂ pounds butternut squash, peeled, seeded, cut into ³/₄-inch cubes
> 1 cup low sodium beef broth
> 1 teaspoon honey

1. In a shallow baking dish, combine sherry, soy sauce, and lemon juice. Add pork slices, turning or stirring to coat the pork, cover dish, and refrigerate mixture for at least 30 minutes.

2. Coat a nonstick skillet with cooking spray, heat, and brown pork, reserving marinade. Add 1 teaspoon oil, and when the oil is heated, add the squash and cook, stirring, for about 1 minute.

3. Add broth, reserved marinade, and honey, bring mixture to a boil, reduce heat, and simmer for 10 minutes or until the pork is cooked through and squash is tender. Serve hot.

SERVES 4

APPROXIMATELY 55.0 MILLIGRAMS CHOLESTEROL PER SERVING

◆ ◆ ◆ ◆

VEAL BIRDS
IN TOMATO SOUR-CREAM SAUCE

▶ ▶

Veal is relatively low in fat compared to other meats. However, 4 ounces of roasted lean veal contain an average of 120 milligrams of cholesterol, while there is an average of 100 milligrams for beef, lamb, and pork. That is why this dish has been designed to make a small amount of veal go a long way.

Veal birds, known as *oiseaux sans tête* in France, are thin cutlets that are stuffed and rolled and served with a sauce. Here, the veal is pounded superthin, stuffed with a savory blend of escarole and bread crumbs, and served with a tomato and sour cream (mock, of course) sauce.

4   *boneless veal cutlets, ¼ inch thick (about 2½*
    ounces
    each)
2   *teaspoons vegetable oil*
    Vegetable oil cooking spray
1   *small onion, minced*
1   *clove garlic, finely minced*
1   *small stalk celery, finely diced*
6   *ounces fresh escarole, trimmed, rinsed, drained,*
    and chopped
1   *tablespoon dry white wine or white wine vinegar*
1   *teaspoon Worcestershire sauce*
1   *cup fine bread crumbs, preferably homemade*
    from dry French bread

Salt and pepper to taste
2 *teaspoons grated Parmesan cheese*
$1/2$ *cup low sodium chicken broth*
$1/3$ *cup low sodium tomato sauce*
$1/3$ *cup Mock Sour Cream (page 3)*
3 *tablespoons minced fresh parsley*

1. Place veal cutlets between sheets of plastic wrap and flatten to a thickness of about $1/8$ inch. Set aside.

2. Heat oil in a heavy skillet coated with cooking spray. Add onion, garlic, and celery and cook over medium heat, stirring often, for 5 minutes. Add escarole, wine, and Worcestershire sauce and cook, stirring often, for an additional 5 minutes or until escarole is limp. Remove from heat and transfer contents of skillet with a slotted spoon to a mixing bowl to cool slightly. Do not wipe out skillet.

3. Add bread crumbs, rosemary, and salt and pepper to escarole mixture. If mixture seems too dry, moisten with 1 or 2 tablespoons of the broth. Stir to blend ingredients thoroughly.

4. Divide escarole mixture among the cutlets and sprinkle each with $1/2$ teaspoon of the grated cheese. Fold over about $1/2$ inch of long sides of cutlets, then roll up from the short side and tie at each end with kitchen string.

5. Place rolls in the skillet, adding additional cooking spray if needed, and cook over medium-high heat, turning to brown all sides. Transfer rolls to a bowl and set aside.

6. Add remaining broth to skillet and stir over high heat until mixture simmers. Reduce heat, stir in tomato sauce, and return veal rolls and any accumulated juices from bowl to skillet. Cover and simmer over very low heat for about 10 minutes or until veal is tender. Using tongs, transfer veal to a heated serving platter.

7. Add Mock Sour Cream and 2 tablespoons of the parsley to sauce in skillet. Stir over very low heat for 1 minute or until sauce is heated through. Do not boil. Spoon 2 or 3 tablespoons of sauce over veal, sprinkle with remaining parsley, and serve with rest of sauce on the side.

SERVES 4

APPROXIMATELY 57.0 MILLIGRAMS CHOLESTEROL PER SERVING

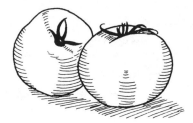

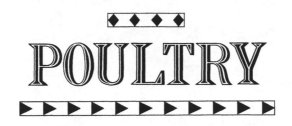

POULTRY

◆ ◆ ◆ ◆ ◆

TANDOORI CHICKEN

▶ ▶

I ndian food is currently enjoying a groundswell of popularity throughout this country, and I believe justifiably so. One need only enter a good Indian restaurant to be seduced by the dizzying bouquet of aromas.

Tandoori cooking is a most agreeable introduction to the vast and intricate cuisine of India. The tandoor is a clay oven with a coal or wood fire. For preparation, chicken, meat, fish, or bread is placed in the tandoor, which is open at the top with a fire blazing inside. The foods are thus magnificently roasted. Chicken, which the Indians invariably skin, is traditionally marinated in yogurt, herbs, and spices before being cooked. The result is tender and juicy chicken, redolent of the various spices and herbs in which it has been marinated.

It is customary to serve tandoori chicken with seasoned, dry-fried onions and lemon wedges, along with basmati rice pilaf, *dal* (a mild lentil dish), *raita* (yogurt with chopped cucumbers and mint), and assorted chutneys. But do give my version a try with Turmeric Rice (page 151) or Wild Rice with Tipsy Currants (page 149).

³/₄   cup nonfat plain yogurt
¹/₂   teaspoon freshly grated ginger root or ¹/₄ teaspoon
      powdered
1   large clove garlic, finely minced
¹/₂   teaspoon hot paprika, or to taste
1¹/₄ teaspoons ground coriander

1¼   teaspoons ground cumin
½   teaspoon ground turmeric
¼   teaspoon cardamom
1½   tablespoons finely minced yellow onion
½   teaspoon black pepper
     Juice of 1 average lime
2   pounds chicken breasts with bone, skinned,
     halved, and trimmed of all visible fat

1. Combine all ingredients, except the chicken, and stir well to blend.
2. Coat the chicken with the marinade, using pressure to rub the spices into the flesh. Cover and refrigerate for 8 hours or overnight.
3. Preheat broiler.
4. Remove chicken from marinade and broil 5 inches from the heat, turning occasionally, for about 35 minutes or until chicken is tender.

SERVES 4
APPROXIMATELY 86.0 MILLIGRAMS CHOLESTEROL PER SERVING

◆ ◆ ◆ ◆ ◆

BRAISED CHICKEN THIGHS
WITH APRICOTS AND PEACHES

▶ ▶

Braising is a two-step method of cooking meats or vegetables in which the food is first browned, then slow-cooked in a small amount of liquid. Not only does braising tenderize foods by gently breaking down their fibers, but the lengthy cooking time allows them to fully develop their flavors.

The result of this unconventional but exquisite coupling of chicken and fruit is a complete and satisfying one-dish meal that needs only a steamed vegetable or a salad to make an unusual and enjoyable dinner.

1	tablespoon olive oil
1³/₄	pounds chicken thighs with bone, skinned and trimmed of all visible fat
1	medium onion, chopped
2	cloves garlic, flattened
¹/₂	cup dry white wine
1	teaspoon dried rosemary, crumbled
1	cup rice
2	cups water
1	tablespoon orange juice
¹/₄	cup dried apricot halves
¹/₄	cup dried peach halves
	Salt and freshly ground pepper to taste

1. Heat oil in a large nonstick skillet and brown chicken over medium-high heat. Remove chicken and keep warm.

2. Reduce heat to medium, add onion and garlic to skillet, and cook until onion is translucent, stirring occasionally.

3. Add wine and rosemary and cook for 1 minute, then return chicken to pan and cover tightly. Simmer for 15 minutes, shaking pan occasionally.

4. Uncover pan, pour rice in around chicken thighs, and cook rice briefly, stirring to coat. Add water, orange juice, apricots, peaches, and salt and pepper, and stir. Cover and simmer for 20 minutes or until liquid is absorbed and rice is cooked through. Taste and correct seasonings, if desired. Do not stir while rice is cooking.

SERVES 4

APPROXIMATELY 93.0 MILLIGRAMS CHOLESTEROL PER SERVING

♦ ♦ ♦ ♦ ♦

DEVILED CHICKEN DIJON
(Adapted from Alan Litke)

▶ ▶

M y friend Alan is handsome, intelligent, creative, successful, and currently single. He loves to entertain friends and business associates, as well as potential romantic partners.

Alan has been around the butcher block once or twice and, yes, he enjoys cooking, but he refuses to fuss about the kitchen. Give him good, simple, honest fare and he'll present it with style. He introduced me to this wonderful-looking concoction of chicken breasts marinated in a pleasantly spiked bath of cayenne, mustard, wine, parsley, and shallots, then lightly breaded with seasoned crumbs and set to bake to a golden turn.

$1/4$ cup plus 2 tablespoons fresh lemon juice
$1/4$ cup Chablis or other fruity white wine
3 tablespoons Dijon mustard
$1/4$ cup chopped fresh parsley
2 large shallots, minced
$1/4$ teaspoon cayenne, or to taste
2 whole boneless, skinless chicken breasts (about 1 pound), halved and trimmed of all visible fat
$1^1/2$ cups fresh bread crumbs, preferably from day-old French bread
Salt and freshly ground pepper to taste
Vegetable oil cooking spray

1. In a large bowl, combine ¼ cup of the lemon juice with wine, mustard, parsley, and shallots. Rub chicken with cayenne and marinate in lemon juice mixture, refrigerated, for at least 4 hours.

2. Preheat oven to 350°F.

3. Place bread crumbs in a shallow bowl and mix with salt and pepper to taste. Press chicken into bread crumb mixture, coating well on all sides. Place breasts on a baking sheet lightly coated with cooking spray and bake for 30 minutes or until golden and crisp outside.

4. Transfer chicken to a heated serving platter, sprinkle with remaining 2 tablespoons lemon juice, and serve.

SERVES 4

APPROXIMATELY 64.0 MILLIGRAMS CHOLESTEROL PER SERVING

◆◆◆◆◆

CHICKEN FRICASSEE
WITH PEPPERS AND ONIONS

▶ ▶

Chicken fricassee is an old favorite of mine. I can remember my mother's preparation, sautéed in butter, of course, stewed with vegetables, wine, and herbs, thickened with cream, and served with buttered noodles. It just didn't get better than that!

In my teens I was eating a lighter version: Chicken Cacciatore, a wonderful Italian-American creation consisting of chicken pieces, mushrooms, onions, various herbs and spices, and wine. *Cacciatore* is the Italian word for "hunter," and so in the ensuing years whenever I saw "chicken hunter style" on the menu, I always ordered what I knew would be the cook's version of good old fricassee.

In my Good-Eating rendition, just-browned chicken braises in wine and herbs, then stews to perfection with select vegetables.

　1　*3-pound chicken, skinned, trimmed of all visible*
　　　fat, and cut into 8 serving pieces
　　　Olive oil cooking spray
　2　*teaspoons olive oil*
　2　*large onions, sliced*
1¹/₂　*cups dry white wine*
　2　*tablespoons chopped fresh parsley*
¹/₂　*teaspoon dried thyme or 2 teaspoons chopped*
　　　fresh

1   teaspoon fennel seeds
1   large stalk celery, sliced thin
2   medium green bell peppers, seeded and cut into thin strips
1   medium red bell pepper, seeded and cut into thin strips
½   pound mushrooms, wiped clean, trimmed, and sliced
1   pound large fresh tomatoes, peeled and chopped, with juice
    Salt and freshly ground pepper to taste

1. Preheat oven to 300°F.

2. In a medium ovenproof stockpot or casserole with a tight-fitting lid, brown chicken in cooking spray and oil over medium-high heat, turning once or twice, until golden. Remove chicken, reduce heat to medium, add onions, and sauté until wilted. Add 1 or 2 tablespoons of wine if mixture is very dry and sticking to pot.

3. When onion is wilted, return chicken to pot and add 1 cup wine, parsley, thyme, and fennel seeds. Cover, transfer pot to preheated oven, and bake for 1 hour.

4. Add celery, bell peppers, mushrooms, tomatoes, and remaining wine to casserole, cover and return to oven for 30 minutes or until chicken is very tender. Taste and add salt and pepper, if desired. Serve chicken with vegetables from the pot.

SERVES 4

APPROXIMATELY 104.0 MILLIGRAMS CHOLESTEROL PER SERVING

◆◆◆◆◆

ORIENTAL CHICKEN ROLLS

▶▶▶▶▶▶▶▶▶▶▶▶▶▶▶▶▶▶▶▶▶▶▶▶▶▶

O ne of the many splendid Japanese creations I admire is *nagimi*, a simply composed dish of thin-sliced chicken that has been marinated in a fragrant "master blend" of soy, sugar, ginger, garlic, and sake, fitted with various vegetables, then rolled up and secured with a wooden toothpick for a brief browning in the skillet. To finish, the rolls are cooked until tender in a mixture of marinade and broth. For presentation, the nagimi is brought to the table on a bed of lettuce, cradled in a beautifully hand-painted lacquer tray.

My version is a reasonable facsimile of classic nagimi, one that will be as fragrant, flavorful, and attractive as the original. Transfer the cooked chicken rolls from the skillet, divide among four heated serving plates, and top with the remaining sauce. Rice is the natural choice to serve with this dish, as is a salad of shredded zucchini and yellow squash.

2   teaspoons sugar
2   tablespoons low sodium soy sauce
2   tablespoons white wine or sake
1   teaspoon freshly grated ginger root
1   medium clove garlic, minced
2   whole boneless, skinless chicken breasts (about 1
    pound), halved and trimmed of all visible fat
1   medium carrot
6   scallions, white and tender greens
    Vegetable oil cooking spray

1   *tablespoon peanut oil*
$^1/_2$ *cup low sodium chicken broth*

1. Combine sugar, soy sauce, wine, ginger root, and garlic in a dish large enough to hold the chicken in one layer.

2. Cut each chicken breast half into two equal pieces and add to dish, turning to coat all sides. Cover and refrigerate for at least 1 hour.

3. Cut carrot into matchstick-size strips about 3 inches in length and blanch in boiling water for 30 seconds. Drain and set aside.

4. Remove chicken from dish and reserve any leftover marinade. Place chicken on a sheet of wax paper and gently pound pieces into rectangular shapes of even thickness.

5. Cut scallions in half lengthwise and then into 3-inch lengths, or of a size to fit lengthwise onto chicken pieces. Divide scallions and carrot matchsticks equally among the eight chicken pieces. Carefully roll up chicken pieces to enclose vegetables and secure with string or toothpicks.

6. Heat cooking spray and peanut oil in a nonstick skillet large enough to hold all the rolls. Brown rolls on all sides over medium heat. Remove chicken from skillet and drain off any excess oil.

7. Raise heat, add broth and any reserved marinade to skillet. Cook, swirling pan constantly, until hot and bubbly and slightly reduced.

8. Lower heat and return chicken rolls to skillet, turning with tongs to coat with liquid. Cover and cook over medium-low heat for 10 minutes or until chicken is tender and cooked through.

SERVES 4

APPROXIMATELY 66.0 MILLIGRAMS CHOLESTEROL PER SERVING

◆ ◆ ◆ ◆ ◆

APPLE-GLAZED CHICKEN

▶ ▶

This tangy marinade serves three purposes. First, its delightful flavors are thoroughly absorbed by the chicken in the soaking process. Next, because the marinade contains acids (vinegar and lemon juice) and herbs (thyme and rosemary), it tenderizes the fibers cf the chicken. Third, the apple juice mixture produces a thin, glossy coating, a glaze as it were, for a most attractive presentation.

> 3   tablespoons thawed frozen apple juice concentrate
> 2   tablespoons honey
> 1/4 cup cider vinegar
> 2   tablespoons prepared Dijon mustard
>   Juice of one large lemon
> 1/8 teaspoon cayenne pepper, or more to taste
> 1   teaspoon chopped fresh thyme or 1/2 teaspoon
>   dried
> 1/2 teaspoon crushed fresh or dried rosemary
> 1/4 teaspoon salt, or to taste
> 2   pounds chicken breasts with bone, skinned,
>   halved, and trimmed of all visible fat
>   Vegetable oil cooking spray
>   Fresh thyme or rosemary sprigs for garnish

1. In a shallow baking dish, combine apple juice concentrate, honey, vinegar, mustard, lemon juice, cayenne, herbs, and salt if desired. Add chicken, turning to coat well, cover, and refrigerate for at least 2 hours.

2. Preheat oven to 350°F.

3. Remove chicken and marinade from dish, reserving marinade. Wipe out dish and coat lightly with cooking spray. Return chicken pieces to dish in a single layer and bake for about 35 minutes or until tender, brushing frequently with marinade. Transfer chicken to a heated platter or individual serving dishes, garnish with herb sprigs if desired, and serve.

SERVES 4
APPROXIMATELY 85.0 MILLIGRAMS CHOLESTEROL
   PER SERVING

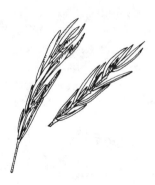

◆◆◆◆◆

HOT AND COOL CHICKEN SKEWERS

▶▶▶▶▶▶▶▶▶▶▶▶▶▶▶▶▶▶▶▶▶▶▶▶▶▶▶

M y early memories of food cooked on the outdoor grill bring mixed feelings of horror and delight. I remember once-juicy hamburgers mercilessly charred to ashes, gorgeous hunks of sirloin curled up at the edges and drained of color and flavor, hot dogs that became shriveled swizzle sticks, and potatoes reduced to empty shells. Nonetheless, everything was always eaten with relish—or with ketchup, mustard, mayonnaise, or anything else that could mask the textures of the burnt offerings.

If there is one lesson I've learned from those early experiences it is this: good cooks pay attention. This chicken should be moist and tender but cooked through (to guard against salmonella), and the grilling or broiling process, which takes only a few minutes to complete, should be closely watched.

2   *whole boneless, skinless, chicken breasts (about 1 pound), halved and trimmed of all visible fat*
1   *tablespoon fresh lime juice*
1   *tablespoon dry white wine*
1   *teaspoon olive oil*
¹/₄   *teaspoon cayenne, or to taste*
¹/₂   *teaspoon sweet paprika*
¹/₄   *teaspoon dried oregano*
¹/₄   *teaspoon dried thyme*
¹/₄   *teaspoon salt, or to taste*
   Freshly ground pepper to taste
2   *cloves garlic, pressed*

2   small shallots, finely minced or pressed
4   tablespoons Herbed Yogurt Dip (page 26), or to
     taste

1. Rinse chicken, pat dry, and cut each breast half into 6 equal pieces.

2. Combine remaining ingredients, except yogurt dip, toss chicken pieces in marinade, cover, and refrigerate for at least 2 hours.

3. Prepare grill or preheat broiler.

4. Thread chicken pieces equally on 4 skewers (if using bamboo skewers, soak them in water first) and grill 4 to 5 inches from heat source, turning occasionally, for about 5 minutes per side or until just cooked through.

5. Divide among 4 plates and serve with Herbed Yogurt Dip.

SERVES 4
APPROXIMATELY 64.0 MILLIGRAMS CHOLESTEROL
    PER SERVING

◆ ◆ ◆ ◆ ◆

CHICKEN WITH GARLIC
AND WILD MUSHROOMS

▶ ▶

For thousands of years garlic has made its presence known like few other foods or flavorings ever savored by man. And for thousands of years man has tried to cope with its so-called alliaceous odor. But cope we do, since there's absolutely no substitute for the uncompromising, vigorous, and sensuous flavor imparted by garlic.

It is paradoxical that the amount of garlic in a dish does not always determine the strength of its flavor; rather, its pungency is determined by the manner in which the garlic is prepared. Whole baked garlic, as it's used in this recipe, will produce a sweet, nutlike flavor and, as an unexpected bonus, will leave little or no garlic odor on your breath.

A recipe to excite the palate and satisfy the soul, this dish combines three of the world's most ancient and treasured foods: the homely, heroic chicken, garlic in great amounts, and earthy, musky, wild mushrooms. Serve it with something uncomplicated like noodles or orzo and peas.

1   head garlic, papery outer layer removed
1   tablespoon walnut oil or olive oil
2   whole boneless, skinless chicken breasts (about 1
     pound), halved and trimmed of all visible fat
3   tablespoons mildly sweet white wine (such as
     Sauternes)
³/₄   cup low sodium chicken broth

$^1/_2$ *pound wild mushrooms (shiitake, chanterelle,*
oyster, or other fresh mushrooms), wiped clean
and stemmed, larger mushrooms cut in half
Salt and freshly ground pepper to taste

1. Preheat oven (I use the toaster oven) to 375°F.
2. Place garlic head on a sheet of aluminum foil and bring foil up to enclose garlic completely but loosely. Bake for 1 hour. Remove from oven and cool slightly. When cool enough to handle, separate cloves and pinch each clove to release garlic from skin. Discard skins and set roasted garlic aside.
3. Heat walnut or olive oil in large nonstick skillet over medium heat. Add chicken and brown, turning once or twice. Remove chicken from skillet and keep warm.
4. Raise heat to medium-high and add wine, swirling skillet quickly to deglaze. Add broth and simmer until mixture is reduced by about one-third.
5. Lower heat to medium-low, add mushrooms and roasted garlic to skillet along with reserved chicken, cover and pan-roast gently, shaking pan occasionally, for about 10 minutes or until chicken is cooked through. Taste and add salt and pepper, if desired.

SERVES 4
APPROXIMATELY 65.0 MILLIGRAMS CHOLESTEROL
    PER SERVING

◆◆◆◆◆

CHICKEN IN LEMON YOGURT
WITH PEAS AND ARTICHOKES

▶ ▶

I had an aunt who derived an inordinate amount of pleasure from shocking her nearest and dearest. Nothing major, just small, nittering things, subtle but deadly. Like injecting salty language into otherwise innocent conversations. Or mimicking expressions of others to their faces. Things like that. The one I loathed most was her lemon trick. She would cut a plump, juicy lemon in half and suck on it, extracting every last drop of its liquor. I would stare at this daring feat, feeling my lips start to furl, slowly tightening into a full pucker. She would dare me to duplicate this act, knowing full well I lacked the courage.

These days I *love* lemon, despite my aunt and her hijinks, and lemon plays a pivotal role in this recipe. Not only does it help tenderize the chicken, its lovely tart sweetness flavors the smooth and creamy yogurt sauce.

Blending cornstarch with the yogurt and adding a few teaspoons of the hot cooking liquid helps keep the yogurt from breaking down when cooked.

Vegetable oil cooking spray
2 *teaspoons vegetable oil*
4 *chicken legs with thighs (about 2 pounds), skinned, trimmed of all visible fat, and separated at the joint*
2 *medium leeks, white and tender greens, well rinsed and chopped*

2   large cloves garlic, minced
1   cup low sodium chicken broth
    Juice of one large lemon (3 to 4 tablespoons)
1/8 teaspoon ground nutmeg
1/4 teaspoon dried summer savory or thyme, crushed
1   cup frozen petite peas, thawed
2   cups frozen or canned and drained, water-packed
    artichoke hearts, cut in half
1   tablespoon cornstarch
1/2 cup low fat plain yogurt
    Salt to taste

1. Heat cooking spray and oil in a nonstick skillet. Add chicken and brown on all sides over medium heat, removing pieces as they brown. When all chicken has been removed, add leeks and garlic to skillet and cook until leeks are softened. Add 1 or 2 tablespoons of broth if leeks are dry and sticking to the pan.

2. Add broth, lemon juice, nutmeg, and summer savory, and cook over medium heat for 5 minutes. Return chicken to skillet, cover, and simmer for 20 minutes. Add peas and artichokes and cook for an additional 10 minutes. Remove from heat.

3. Blend cornstarch with yogurt, add a little hot liquid from skillet, and stir well. Add mixture to skillet and cook over very low heat, stirring well to combine flavors and heat sauce through. Do not boil. Taste and correct seasonings, adding additional lemon juice if desired.

SERVES 4

APPROXIMATELY 108.0 MILLIGRAMS CHOLESTEROL

PER SERVING

◆◆◆◆◆

TURKEY CHILI

▶ ▶

The secret to a more flavorful chili is to use the freshest, best quality chili powder you can find (it stays fresh longer if refrigerated after opening). And cooking the dish covered helps keep the turkey moist and tender.

1	tablespoon olive oil
1	cup coarsely chopped red onion
2	large cloves garlic, minced
$^1/_2$	tablespoon ground cumin
2	tablespoons chili powder
1	35-ounce can no-salt-added plum tomatoes in puree, coarsely chopped
1	pound turkey white meat cutlets, cut into large, bite-size pieces
1	medium green bell pepper, diced
$^1/_2$	teaspoon dried oregano
$^1/_2$	teaspoon hot red pepper flakes, or to taste
3	cups cooked or canned, rinsed, and drained red kidney beans
2	tablespoons minced fresh cilantro or parsley
	Salt and freshly ground pepper to taste

1. Heat oil over medium heat in large stockpot and sauté onion and garlic, stirring frequently, until onion is translucent.

2. Sprinkle cumin and chili powder over onion mixture and stir quickly to dissolve.

3. Raise heat to medium-high and add tomatoes with

puree, turkey pieces, green pepper, oregano, and hot pepper flakes. Stir well to combine ingredients.

4. When mixture just comes to a boil, cover, reduce heat, and simmer gently, stirring occasionally, for 1 hour.

5. Add kidney beans and cilantro or parsley, cover, and continue to cook for an additional 30 minutes. Taste and season with salt and pepper, if desired.

SERVES 8
APPROXIMATELY 36.0 MILLIGRAMS CHOLESTEROL
PER SERVING

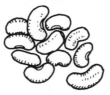

◆◆◆◆◆

MUSHROOM-STUFFED TURKEY IN WINE SAUCE

▶ ▶

This dish fits nicely into any menu, whether simple or flamboyant. And because there is almost no vegetable that will clash with turkey rolls, experiment with the accompaniments.

4   teaspoons olive oil
     Olive oil cooking spray
1   large clove garlic, chopped
2   large shallots or ¹/₂ onion, chopped
1   cup sliced mushrooms
2   tablespoons chopped fresh Italian parsley
8   turkey breast cutlets (about 1¹/₄ pounds),
     pounded thin
¹/₂ cup dry white wine
¹/₄ cup low sodium chicken broth
1   tablespoon lemon juice
     Salt and freshly ground pepper to taste

1. Heat 2 teaspoons oil in a large nonstick skillet coated with cooking spray. Add garlic, shallots, and mushrooms and cook over medium heat, stirring occasionally, until mushrooms are tender.

2. Remove from heat, reserve 2 heaping tablespoons of the mushroom mixture, and stir parsley into remainder.

3. Spread parsleyed mushroom mixture from skillet over the cutlets to within ¹/₂ inch of the edges and roll tightly,

securing each roll with string or a wooden toothpick inserted diagonally so that the rolls can be turned in the skillet.

4. Wipe skillet, heat remaining 2 teaspoons oil, and brown the rolls over medium heat, turning occasionally. Remove rolls to a platter.

5. Raise heat and add wine, broth, lemon juice, and salt and pepper to taste. Bring to a boil and cook for 2 minutes. Reduce heat and return rolls and reserved mushroom mixture to skillet, turning each roll to coat with liquid. Cover skillet, and simmer over low heat for about 10 minutes or until turkey is cooked through. Serve with sauce from the skillet.

SERVES 4

APPROXIMATELY 90.0 MILLIGRAMS CHOLESTEROL
    PER SERVING

◆◆◆◆◆

TURKEY CUTLETS WITH LEMON, CAPERS, AND SAGE

▶ ▶

I've already discussed elsewhere in my Good Eating Series my passion for the sauce known as *grenobloise*, which is prepared in the style of Grenoble, France. Traditionally, it is made with slightly browned butter to which capers and lemon are added. Fabulous with fish, grenobloise is also magnificent with poultry in general and with these turkey cutlets in particular.

For this recipe, grenobloise is made even more delectable with the help of that wonderful little old herbaceous turkey-helper, sage. In addition, this sauce eliminates the once-mandatory half cup of butter and uses a touch of olive oil instead.

Small new potatoes boiled in their jackets, along with glazed carrots or petit pois, are wonderful companions for the turkey. A Barley and Mushroom Casserole (page 155) and Butternut Squash with Brown Sugar Glaze (page 171) might also make interesting side dishes.

1¹/₂   *tablespoons olive oil*
1   *clove garlic, flattened*
8   *turkey breast cutlets (about 1¹/₄ pounds),*
   flattened to ¹/₄ inch thick (pound gently or they
   may split apart)
   Superfine flour
1   *large lemon*
¹/₂   *cup dry white wine*

2   teaspoons capers, rinsed and drained
1   large sprig fresh sage, chopped, plus 4 sprigs for
    garnish

1. Heat oil in a large nonstick skillet over medium-low heat. Add garlic and sauté, stirring frequently, until softened.
2. Dredge turkey cutlets lightly in flour, shaking to remove any excess. Raise heat to medium and quickly sauté cutlets, shaking pan, until lightly browned on both sides. Remove and keep warm.
3. Cut lemon in half. Raise heat to medium-high and squeeze juice into pan. Press lemon, cut side down, into pan and rub around to extract any remaining juice. Pour in wine and add capers and sage and cook, swirling pan continuously, for about 4 minutes or until slightly reduced. Remove lemon halves.
4. Return cutlets to pan and sauté for 2 minutes, turning cutlets once to coat with glaze. Serve garnished with fresh sage leaves.

SERVES 4
APPROXIMATELY 90.0 MILLIGRAMS CHOLESTEROL
    PER SERVING

◆◆◆◆◆

SWEET AND SPICY TURKEY WITH POLENTA

▶ ▶

Somewhere between picadillo and Sloppy Joes, this dish has a spicy sauce that marries very well with the sensible polenta. Serve with a crispy salad of romaine lettuce.

1	teaspoon vegetable oil
1¹/₂	pounds light meat turkey, ground
1	medium onion, chopped
1	large clove garlic, minced
1¹/₂	cups low sodium tomato sauce
1	small jalapeño pepper, seeded and diced (wear rubber gloves), or to taste
¹/₂	teaspoon dried oregano
2	teaspoons sugar
¹/₄	teaspoon ground cinnamon
¹/₂	teaspoon ground cumin
	Pinch ground cloves
¹/₂	cup red wine
¹/₄	teaspoon salt, or to taste
	Basic Polenta (page 157)

1. Heat oil in a large nonstick skillet over medium heat and cook turkey, breaking up any clumps with a wooden spoon, until it loses its raw color. Add onion and garlic and cook until onion is soft and turkey is browned.

2. Add remaining ingredients, except salt and polenta, bring to a boil, reduce heat, and barely simmer for 20 minutes. Taste and add salt, if desired.

---

3. If polenta is cold, reheat it in a low (300°F.) oven for 15 minutes or briefly in a microwave, then cut into six squares. Place squares in the center of warmed soup plates and spoon turkey mixture over polenta.

SERVES 6
APPROXIMATELY 75.0 MILLIGRAMS CHOLESTEROL
PER SERVING

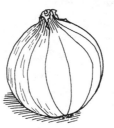

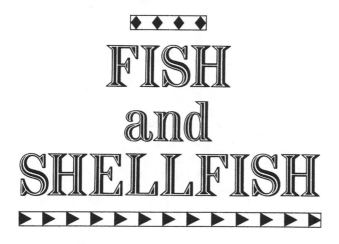

FISH
and
SHELLFISH

◆ ◆ ◆ ◆ ◆

SPINACH-STUFFED COD STEAKS

▶ ▶

Whenever you see *à la Florentine* listed on the menu, you can be sure that the dish will be presented on a bed of, or topped with, spinach—often in concert with a freight-load of artery-clogging Mornay sauce.

Here is a streamlined version of the dish the French call *Cabillaud à la Florentine*; that is, "cod in the style of Florence," Italy. My dish teams the codfish with vegetables, herbs, spices, and wine—and the mandatory verdant spinach. The results are a dish that is attractive, succulent, and flavorful, requiring nothing more than appreciative dinner companions with whom to share the experience.

10	ounces fresh spinach, trimmed and well rinsed
2	teaspoons olive oil
3	tablespoons finely chopped onion
2	medium cloves garlic, minced
1	tablespoon chopped scallions, white and tender greens
1	tablespoon chopped fresh parsley
1/2	large lemon, divided in half
	Salt and freshly ground pepper to taste
	Vegetable oil cooking spray
4	cod steaks (about 1 1/4 pounds)
1/4	cup dry white wine or vermouth

1. Preheat oven to 350°F.

2. In a large pot, steam spinach, stirring occasionally, until well wilted.

---

3. Meanwhile, heat oil in a nonstick skillet. Add onion, garlic, and scallions and cook over medium heat, stirring often, until onion is translucent but not brown.

4. Remove spinach from pot, squeeze out as much liquid as possible, and chop. Add spinach to onion mixture and combine well. Stir in the juice of ¼ lemon and add salt and pepper to taste. Cook briefly over medium heat, stirring, to blend flavors.

5. Spray the bottom of a baking dish large enough to hold the fish in one layer with cooking oil. Lay steaks in the dish, mound ¼ of the spinach filling in the hollow between the tails of each steak, and secure tail ends with a wooden toothpick. (If the steaks do not have tails, make a cut from the side into the middle of each steak, open the cut gently to expose a "pie slice," and squeeze filling into the opening. Secure with a toothpick, if necessary.) Pour wine or vermouth around steaks.

6. Sprinkle fish with juice of the remaining lemon, cover with foil, and bake for 10 minutes. Remove foil and bake for an additional 5 minutes or until fish is cooked through and filling is steaming.

SERVES 4

APPROXIMATELY 61.0 MILLIGRAMS CHOLESTEROL PER SERVING

◆ ◆ ◆ ◆ ◆

BAKED SEA BASS
WITH SHALLOTS AND CAPERS

▶ ▶

$\mathbb{S}$ea bass is a fish of incomparable tenderness and moistness. It is considered of such high quality, in fact, that it is frequently served raw as sushi or sashimi. I adore it presented in this fashion: baked and sauced with a truly heavenly blend of wine, lemon, shallots, and capers.

Keep an eye on the bass as it bakes. I feel it's better to remove the fish from the oven just before it's fully cooked (perhaps somewhere between 8 and 10 minutes for this recipe) as it will continue cooking in the baking dish.

1¼	pounds sea bass fillets
1	tablespoon fresh lemon juice
	Salt and freshly ground pepper to taste
	Vegetable oil cooking spray
2	teaspoons unsalted margarine
2	large shallots, finely minced
1	cup dry white wine
1	tablespoon minced fresh parsley or ½ tablespoon dried
1½	tablespoons capers, rinsed and drained

1. Preheat oven to 350°F.

2. Sprinkle both sides of sea bass with lemon juice and salt and pepper to taste. Place fish in a shallow baking pan coated with cooking spray and set aside.

3. Melt margarine in a nonstick skillet. Add shallots and sauté over low heat, stirring often, for 5 minutes. Raise heat

---

Fish and Shellfish ◆ 107

to medium and add wine, parsley, and capers, stirring until wine just starts to simmer. Pour contents of skillet over sea bass.

4. Bake for 8 to 10 minutes or until fish is just cooked through. Serve immediately.

SERVES 4

APPROXIMATELY 58.0 MILLIGRAMS CHOLESTEROL PER SERVING

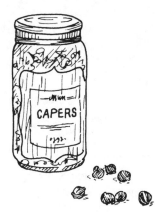

◆ ◆ ◆ ◆ ◆

GRILLED SWORDFISH
WITH MELON CUCUMBER RELISH

▶ ▶

My first experience with a melon relish was one warm summer evening on the patio of a tiny restaurant in the Virgin Islands. The combination of flavors and colors was so refreshing, I felt compelled to create a version of my own. The restaurant, unfortunately, is long gone and the name forgotten, but that dish remains fresh in my mind.

$^1/_2$ cup fruity white wine, such as Chablis
  3 tablespoons fresh lime juice
  2 generous dashes hot pepper sauce, or to taste
  1 large clove garlic, pressed
  4 swordfish steaks, 1 inch thick (about 5 ounces each)
$^1/_2$ cup finely diced sweet, firm cantaloupe
$^1/_2$ cup finely diced sweet honeydew or canary melon
  1 small cucumber, peeled, seeded, and finely diced
  1 tablespoon fresh lemon juice
  2 teaspoons chopped fresh mint leaves
  1 tablespoon chopped fresh chervil (optional)
  2 teaspoons canola or other light vegetable oil
     Salt and freshly ground pepper to taste

1. Combine wine, 2 tablespoons lime juice, hot pepper sauce, and garlic in a shallow baking dish large enough to hold the fish in one layer. Add fish and turn once to coat with marinade. Cover and refrigerate for 15 to 30 minutes.

2. In a small bowl, combine remaining lime juice with melons, cucumber, lemon juice, mint, chervil, and oil. Stir to blend and refrigerate until ready to serve.

3. Prepare grill and coat lightly with cooking spray, or preheat broiler.

4. Grill or broil swordfish for about 5 minutes per side, turning once and brushing with any reserved marinade.

5. Transfer swordfish to heated serving dishes or a platter, sprinkle with salt and pepper, and serve accompanied by chilled melon-cucumber relish.

SERVES 4

APPROXIMATELY 55.0 MILLIGRAMS CHOLESTEROL PER SERVING

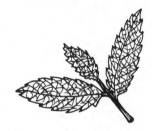

◆ ◆ ◆ ◆ ◆

STEAMED HALIBUT

▶ ▶

Here's a dandy showcase for halibut, which in my opinion is one of the most underrated, overlooked delicacies in all of fishdom. Steaming is a terrific way to treat halibut, and almost any other fish. Cooking this way will, to my mind, retain the shape, essence, and texture of the fish better than any other method of preparation.

However, since steaming seems to hasten the cooking process, keep your eye on the fish, not on the clock.

        1   tablespoon peanut or sesame oil
       10   scallions, white and tender greens, thinly sliced
        1   tablespoon minced fresh ginger root
        1   tablespoon low sodium soy sauce
      ¹/₄   cup dry white wine
        4   halibut steaks, 1¹/₂ inches thick (about 1¹/₂
             pounds)

1. Heat oil in a nonstick skillet. Add scallions and sauté over medium-low heat, stirring often, for about 3 minutes or until scallions are wilted. Stir in ginger and soy sauce, then raise heat, add wine, and bring to a boil. Reduce heat and simmer for 4 minutes. Cover and keep warm.

2. Prepare bamboo steamer or fish steamer (if you don't have a steamer, use a kettle with a large vegetable steamer or a rack lined with cheesecloth, and add water to a depth of 1 inch).

3. When water boils, add fish to steamer. Cover and

---

steam for about 10 minutes, checking after 5 minutes, or until fish is just cooked through.

4. Carefully transfer fish to a heated serving platter and top with scallion sauce.

SERVES 4
APPROXIMATELY 55.0 MILLIGRAMS CHOLESTEROL PER SERVING

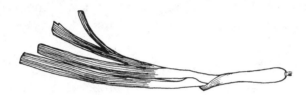

◆ ◆ ◆ ◆ ◆

HALIBUT AND MUSSELS IN TOMATO SAUCE

▶ ▶

You could say I created this dish just for the halibut! Steamed in a lightly aromatic blend of tomatoes and seasonings, this fragrant and flavorful dish is presented with those glorious denizens of the deep—mussels.

¹/₂	tablespoon olive oil
1	clove garlic, chopped
1	28-ounce can no-salt-added plum tomatoes, chopped, with juice
¹/₄	teaspoon hot red pepper flakes, or to taste
	Salt and freshly ground pepper to taste
¹/₂	cup dry white wine
16	mussels, scrubbed and debearded
1	pound halibut fillets, divided into four equal pieces if possible
¹/₄	cup coarsely chopped fresh Italian parsley

1. Heat oil in a large pot or deep skillet and sauté garlic until pale golden.

2. Add tomatoes with their juice, hot pepper and salt if desired, and a few grindings of pepper. Raise heat to medium-high and simmer, stirring occasionally, for about 10 minutes.

3. Add wine and drop the mussels into the pot. Cover and cook for 1 minute.

4. Push the mussels to the sides of the pot, reduce heat, and carefully lay the halibut fillets into the sauce, skin side

---

down. Spoon a little sauce over the fish to moisten it, cover, and barely simmer for 5 to 7 minutes or until the fish loses its translucency and the mussels have opened (the cooking time will depend on the thickness of the fillets).

5. Carefully lift the fish out of the pot and divide among warmed plates. Spoon some sauce over the fish and arrange 4 mussels on each plate. Sprinkle with parsley and serve remaining sauce separately.

SERVES 4

APPROXIMATELY 52.0 MILLIGRAMS CHOLESTEROL PER SERVING

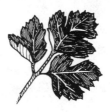

◆ ◆ ◆ ◆ ◆

SWEET AND SOUR FISH

▶ ▶

This appealing recipe combines the classic cooking techniques of steaming and sautéing. The fillets are steam-baked in foil, the greens are steamed, and the scallions and red pepper are sautéed in just a touch of oil. This dish benefits from each cooking method employed: the greens will be just wilted, the baked-in-foil fish will retain its moisture, thus producing a more succulent morsel, and the sauce will deliver a nice blend of sweet and tart flavors.

 1   *pound cod or scrod fillets*
 2   *teaspoons peanut oil*
 4   *scallions, white and tender greens, cut into 2-inch pieces*
 1   *medium red bell pepper, seeded and thinly sliced*
 1   *tablespoon tomato paste*
 1   *teaspoon freshly grated ginger root*
 1   *tablespoon low sodium soy sauce*
 1   *teaspoon sugar*
 ¼   *cup grapefruit juice*
 ¼   *cup low sodium chicken broth*
 ¼   *teaspoon cayenne, or to taste*
 3   *cups steamed, wilted greens, such as chard, spinach, or escarole*

1. Preheat oven to 350°F.
2. Enclose fish fillets in envelopes of baking parchment or foil and bake for 15 minutes.

3. While fish bakes, heat oil in a large nonstick wok or skillet. Add scallion and bell pepper and stir-fry over medium heat for about 2 minutes. Add tomato paste and stir briefly to blend.

4. Add remaining ingredients, except fish and greens, and cook, stirring constantly, for 5 minutes or until liquid is slightly reduced.

5. Arrange greens on a heated serving platter. Remove fish from wrapping and carefully arrange over greens. Spoon contents of skillet over fish and serve.

SERVES 4

APPROXIMATELY 49.0 MILLIGRAMS CHOLESTEROL PER SERVING

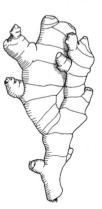

◆◆◆◆◆

HERB-MARINATED TUNA

▶▶▶▶▶▶▶▶▶▶▶▶▶▶▶▶▶▶▶▶▶▶▶▶▶

Whatever your dietary concerns, fish is a winner. Most fish is high in protein and low in fat. In addition, fish provides an ample supply of B vitamins, thiamine, riboflavin, and niacin, and is a natural source of iodine.

High in omega-3, 4 ounces of raw yellowfin tuna has 52 milligrams of cholesterol, 124 calories, 26 grams of protein, and 1.2 grams of fat, making the percentage of calories from fat less than 10 percent. Thus, yellowfin tuna is a pretty good investment on the nutrition market.

In this recipe, the full, rich flavor of the tuna itself is amplified by the infusion of the wonderful Provençale-herb marinade it twice weds.

1/4   cup red wine vinegar
1   tablespoon olive oil
2   garlic cloves, pressed
1/3   teaspoon each: dried oregano, thyme, basil, rosemary, dill seed, and tarragon
1   teaspoon coarsely chopped fresh parsley
1   teaspoon Dijon mustard
    Juice of one large lemon
4   yellowfin tuna steaks (about 1 pound)
1   large lemon, quartered, for garnish

1. Combine vinegar and oil with garlic, herbs, parsley, mustard, and lemon juice in a baking dish or wide bowl large enough to hold the tuna steaks in one layer.

2. Lay the tuna into the marinade, turning once, cover, and refrigerate for 15 to 30 minutes.

3. Prepare grill or preheat broiler.

4. Grill or broil steaks about 5 minutes per side for medium, brushing occasionally with marinade.

5. Transfer to a heated platter and serve garnished with lemon quarters.

SERVES 4

APPROXIMATELY 52.0 MILLIGRAMS CHOLESTEROL PER SERVING

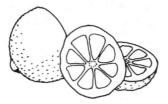

◆ ◆ ◆ ◆ ◆

COLD POACHED RED SNAPPER
WITH HORSERADISH SAUCE

▶ ▶

Fish that is poached is usually done so in *court bouillon*—
fish stock, wine, or a combination of broth and wine—
either in the oven or, as I've indicated here, by simmering
over surface heat. Small whole fish, fillets, and fish steaks
are particularly well suited to either of these poaching
methods.

The poaching liquid I've used here is a highly seasoned court bouillon that imparts its bracing flavor
throughout the flesh of the snapper.

If there is one key to poaching fish it is to keep the
liquid at the simmering point only; if the liquid boils the
fish is almost guaranteed to fall apart.

The horseradish sauce donates a pleasant jolt to the
more subdued delicacy of the snapper. Either bring the fish
platter to the table already sauced, or present the sauce as an
option on the side. Garnish with lemon slices, if desired.

$\frac{1}{2}$ cup finely diced celery
1 cup finely diced carrots
1 cup chopped onion
2 large lemons
1 cup dry white wine
1 bay leaf
6 cups water
1 pound red snapper fillets, divided into 4
   portions
   Dash hot red pepper sauce, or to taste

Salt and coarsely ground pepper to taste
2   *tablespoons light sour cream*
2   *tablespoons nonfat plain yogurt*
1   *tablespoon drained prepared horseradish, or to taste*
2   *tablespoons chopped fresh basil*
4   *large Boston lettuce leaves, rinsed and drained*
4   *large radicchio leaves, rinsed and drained*

1. Prepare poaching liquid by combining celery, carrots, onion, the juice of 1 lemon, wine, bay leaf, and water in a saucepan. Bring to a boil, reduce heat, and simmer gently for 15 minutes.

2. Lay fish fillets into a deep skillet or pot large enough to hold them in one layer. Add enough poaching liquid to barely cover fish. Add hot pepper sauce and salt if desired, and generous grindings of pepper.

3. Cover and simmer very gently for 3 to 5 minutes or until fillets are just cooked through (cooking time will depend on the thickness of the fillets). Transfer fish to a shallow dish and set aside to cool. Strain and reserve poaching liquid.

4. When fish has cooled, add strained poaching liquid to barely cover fillets, seal with plastic wrap and refrigerate for several hours.

5. About 30 minutes before serving, combine sour cream, yogurt, horseradish, juice of the remaining lemon, salt and pepper to taste, and chopped basil. Mix well and chill.

6. Remove fillets from liquid, arrange on a bed of radicchio and Boston lettuce, and serve topped with sauce or with the sauce on the side.

SERVES 4

APPROXIMATELY 44.0 MILLIGRAMS CHOLESTEROL PER SERVING

◆ ◆ ◆ ◆ ◆

MONKFISH FRA DIAVOLO

▶ ▶

Called *lotte* by the French, and bellyfish, frogfish, sea devil, and anglerfish among other apt appellations, monkfish is a large, notoriously unattractive fish. As a saving grace, it is extremely low in fat and cholesterol and boasts a mild, sweet flavor and firm texture that is so reminiscent of lobster it is also known as the poor man's lobster.

This impressive fish is excellent baked, broiled, poached, or braised as it is here. And I find the critter particularly alluring when dressed in the rambunctious Fra Diavolo sauce that is often also associated with lobster.

Serve over a delicate pasta or with steamed rice and a crisp vegetable or salad.

   1   tablespoon olive oil
   3   large cloves garlic, chopped
  ¹/2 cup chopped onion
   2   small, dried hot red peppers or hot red pepper flakes to taste
       Pinch dried oregano
       Pinch dried thyme
  ³/4 cup full-bodied red wine
   1   28-ounce can no-salt-added plum tomatoes in puree, coarsely chopped
  ¹/2 cup diced red bell pepper
   1   tablespoon fresh lemon juice
       Salt and freshly ground pepper to taste
 1¹/2 pounds monkfish fillets, cut into large chunks

1. Heat oil in a large nonstick skillet. Add garlic and onion and sauté over medium heat, stirring often, for 5 minutes or until onion is translucent.

2. Crack open hot peppers and empty seeds into the skillet, discarding pods, or sprinkle with hot pepper flakes. Add oregano, thyme, and wine, and simmer, stirring, for 1 minute.

3. Add tomatoes and their puree, bell pepper, lemon juice, and salt and pepper, and simmer, stirring occasionally, for 20 minutes.

4. Reduce heat, lay fish carefully into sauce, cover, and simmer gently for 15 minutes or until fish is cooked and begins to flake (monkfish has dense flesh and generally requires longer simmering than other fish. Toward the end of the cooking time, test a chunk). Transfer fish to a heated serving platter, top with sauce, and serve.

SERVES 4

APPROXIMATELY 43.0 MILLIGRAMS CHOLESTEROL PER SERVING

◆ ◆ ◆ ◆ ◆

SALMON FILLETS
WITH SCALLION DILL SAUCE

▶ ▶

The wonderful aroma and flavor of fresh dill weed and salmon is true Valhalla, one that simply cannot be duplicated by the coupling of any other fish with fern.

2	teaspoons olive oil
6	scallions, white and tender greens, chopped
1	medium shallot, finely minced
1	cup low sodium chicken broth
	Juice of 1 large lemon
2	tablespoons plus 1 teaspoon chopped fresh dill
	weed or 1 tablespoon plus 1/2 teaspoon dried
	Salt and freshly ground pepper to taste
1	cup water
1	cup dry white wine
6	whole black peppercorns
1/2	small onion, peeled and thinly sliced into rings
4	salmon fillets (about 1 pound)
8	medium bibb lettuce leaves, rinsed and drained
	Fresh dill sprigs for garnish

1. Heat oil in a nonstick skillet. Add scallions and shallot and sauté over medium-low heat, stirring occasionally, for about 5 minutes or until scallions are well wilted.

2. Add broth, lemon juice, and 2 tablespoons fresh or 1 tablespoon dried dill and raise heat to medium-high. Cook for about 5 minutes or until liquid is slightly reduced. Remove from heat and cool slightly.

3. Puree cooled scallion sauce in food processor, taste, and add salt and pepper, if desired. Transfer mixture to a bowl and set aside.

4. Combine water, wine, peppercorns, remaining dill, and onion rings in a deep skillet large enough to hold the salmon in one layer. Bring to a boil, reduce heat, and simmer for 5 minutes. Lay in the fillets, cover, and poach salmon gently for about 5 minutes (cooking time will vary according to the thickness of the fillet and desired degree of doneness. I prefer it moist and just a hint underdone).

5. Arrange 2 lettuce leaves on each of four plates. Arrange fillets over lettuce and spoon sauce over. Garnish each plate with a fresh dill sprig and serve.

SERVES 4

APPROXIMATELY 64.0 MILLIGRAMS CHOLESTEROL PER SERVING

◆ ◆ ◆ ◆ ◆

CHILLED MARINATED SOLE

▶ ▶

Here, the delicate taste of sole gets a lovely wake-up call when allowed to mingle with this fascinating mixture of herbs, lemon, and pepperoncini. Slightly hot, pepperoncini is not a mouth-blazer although it does make its presence known.

Serve well chilled over a bed of shredded radicchio or tender lettuce along with assorted greens for a light and refreshing meal.

$^1/_2$ cup dry white wine

$^1/_2$ cup water

2   tablespoons plus $^1/_4$ cup fresh lemon juice

$^1/_2$ small onion, sliced

6   whole peppercorns

1   bay leaf

1   pound sole fillets, rinsed and patted dry

2   teaspoons olive oil

2   tablespoons drained, chopped pimientos

4   bottled pepperoncini, rinsed, stemmed, and chopped

1   teaspoon chopped fresh thyme or $^1/_2$ teaspoon dried

   Salt to taste

   Radicchio and assorted salad greens

1. In a deep skillet, combine wine, water, 2 tablespoons lemon juice, onion, peppercorns, and bay leaf. Bring to a boil, then reduce heat and simmer for 5 minutes.

---

2. Add sole to skillet and poach gently, uncovered, for 3 minutes or until fish loses its translucency. Carefully remove sole from skillet and set aside to cool. Discard poaching liquid.

3. In a dish large enough to hold the fish, combine remaining ¼ cup lemon juice, olive oil, pimientos, pepperoncini, thyme, and salt to taste. Cut sole into chunks and toss gently in marinade. Cover and chill several hours. Serve on a bed of shredded radicchio and assorted greens.

SERVES 4

APPROXIMATELY 54.0 MILLIGRAMS CHOLESTEROL PER SERVING

◆ ◆ ◆ ◆ ◆

BROILED SEA SCALLOPS
IN TANGERINE SAUCE

▶ ▶

Slightly sweet and curiously "tangy," this unusual combination is absolutely delicious. Although it resembles the lighter, fresher dishes of nouvelle cuisine, this coupling of scallops with fruit is actually more representative of the ancient and honored cuisines of China, Thailand, and India.

If fresh tangerines are not available, substitute a small can of mandarin oranges—preferably packed in juice—and omit the sugar. Serve with the rice of your choice and snow peas.

1   *pound large sea scallops, cut in half*
    Vegetable oil cooking spray
2   *teaspoons sugar*
2   *teaspoons peanut oil*
2   *cloves garlic, finely chopped*
2   *medium shallots, minced*
¹/₄ *cup apple juice*
¹/₄ *cup orange juice*
2   *tangerines, peeled, trimmed, sectioned, and pitted*
1   *teaspoon Worcestershire sauce*
    Salt and freshly ground pepper to taste

1. Preheat broiler.
2. Rinse scallops, pat dry, and arrange in a shallow baking dish lightly coated with cooking spray. Sprinkle sugar over scallops and set aside.

---

3. Heat oil in a nonstick skillet. Add garlic and shallots and sauté over medium-low heat, stirring often, until lightly browned. Add apple and orange juices, tangerine sections, Worcestershire, and salt and pepper to taste. Cook, stirring gently, for 2 minutes.

4. Spoon contents of skillet over scallops in baking pan. Place about 4 inches from heat and broil for 5 minutes or until scallops have lost their translucency and are just cooked through—do not overcook. Transfer to heated serving dishes and serve immediately.

SERVES 4

APPROXIMATELY 38.0 MILLIGRAMS CHOLESTEROL PER SERVING

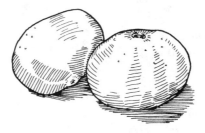

◆ ◆ ◆ ◆ ◆

BAY SCALLOPS STIR-FRIED
WITH CELERY AND WALNUTS

▶ ▶

For this or any other stir-fried preparation, it's best to assemble all your ingredients and complete the chopping, cutting, measuring, and mixing chores in advance of the actual cooking process because stir-frying takes only about eight minutes from start to finish.

Here is a classic Cantonese dish that pays tribute to the great Oriental philosophy of yin and yang: the harmonious blending of opposites. For in this recipe we find crisp (walnuts, celery) and tender (scallops) textures, sweet and sour flavors, and complementing colors that unify to offer one cohesive entity.

1	tablespoon canola or other light vegetable oil
2	medium cloves garlic, thinly sliced
2	large stalks celery, cut diagonally into 1/2-inch slices
4	scallions, white and tender greens, cut diagonally into 1/2-inch slices
1/4	cup walnut pieces
1	pound bay scallops, rinsed and patted dry
1	tablespoon cornstarch
1	cup water
2	teaspoons low sodium soy sauce
2	teaspoons wine vinegar
1/2	teaspoon sugar
	Salt and freshly ground pepper to taste

1. Heat oil in a large nonstick wok or skillet and sauté garlic over medium-high heat until pale golden. Add celery, scallions, and walnuts, and stir for 1 minute.

2. Add scallops to wok and stir for 2 minutes.

3. Dissolve cornstarch in water and stir in soy sauce, vinegar, sugar, and salt and pepper to taste. Pour mixture into wok and stir until sauce thickens. Serve immediately.

SERVES 4

APPROXIMATELY 38.0 MILLIGRAMS CHOLESTEROL PER SERVING

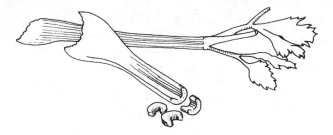

◆ ◆ ◆ ◆ ◆

CLAMS AND MUSSELS MARINARA

▶ ▶

M ollusks are invertebrates with soft bodies covered by a
shell in one or more places. Bivalves are soft-bodied mollusks with two shells hinged together by a strong muscle.
Clams, scallops, oysters, and mussels all fall into this cat-
egory. It sounds almost indecent—even perverted, perhaps—but I have to own up to it: I'm a slave to mollusk
bivalves! I'm crazy for clams and mad for mussels. But all is
not lost, because bivalves are bonkers for me.

Rich in omega-3, they are good, low fat, low cholesterol, low calorie affairs that I enjoy whenever I'm given
the chance. This opportunity knocks twice in my Clams
and Mussels Marinara, thus doubling my pleasure as well.
The marinara sauce is as refreshing as a sea breeze and is
best when sopped up with good crusty bread or ladled
over pasta.

2   teaspoons olive oil
3   large cloves garlic, flattened
¹/₂   cup finely diced carrots
¹/₂   cup finely diced celery
     Pinch oregano
1   teaspoon hot red pepper flakes, or to taste
1   cup dry red wine
1   28-ounce can no-salt-added plum tomatoes in
     puree, chopped
2   dozen littleneck clams, scrubbed
2   dozen mussels, scrubbed and debearded
     Salt and freshly ground pepper to taste

4   large fresh basil leaves, slivered
1   tablespoon fresh lemon juice

1. Heat oil in large, deep nonstick skillet over low flame, and sauté garlic, carrots, and celery, stirring frequently, until garlic begins to turn golden and celery wilts. If garlic becomes very brown, remove with a slotted spoon and discard.

2. Sprinkle with oregano and hot pepper flakes, raise heat to medium-high, and pour in wine and tomatoes. Simmer, stirring occasionally, for 10 minutes or until slightly thickened.

3. Add clams and mussels, cover, reduce heat, and simmer for about 7 minutes or until shells have opened. Taste and add salt and pepper, if desired.

4. Divide clams and mussels among warmed bowls, discarding any that have not opened. Top with sauce, sprinkle with basil slivers and lemon juice, and serve.

SERVES 4

APPROXIMATELY 50.0 MILLIGRAMS CHOLESTEROL PER SERVING

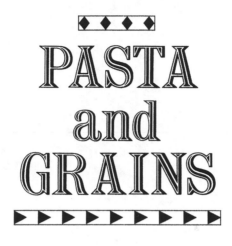

PASTA
and
GRAINS

◆ ◆ ◆ ◆ ◆

FUSILLI WITH FRESH TOMATOES AND MOZZARELLA

▶ ▶

This delicious and fragrant pasta is perfect for steamy summer evenings because the sauce requires no cooking. I prepare this dish when tomatoes are at their ripe, harvest best and fresh basil is readily available.

1	*tablespoon olive oil*
¹/₃	*cup low sodium chicken broth*
3	*large, ripe tomatoes, each cut into eight wedges then cut in half crosswise (do this over a bowl to catch all the juice)*
4	*cloves garlic, flattened slightly*
8 to 10	*fresh basil leaves, cut into thin shreds*
4	*ounces low fat mozzarella, cut into tiny chunks*
	Salt and freshly ground pepper to taste
³/₄	*pound fusilli (corkscrew pasta)*

1. In a large bowl, combine oil, broth, tomatoes with all their juice, garlic, basil, cheese, and salt and pepper and let stand at room temperature for at least 15 minutes, stirring occasionally, to allow flavors to blend. Carefully pick out garlic just before adding pasta.

2. Cook fusilli al dente, drain well, and immediately add hot pasta to the tomato and mozzarella mixture in bowl. Toss gently until the pasta is well coated. The hot pasta will warm

the sauce to a comfortable temperature for summer eating. Ladle into pasta bowls and serve.

SERVES 4
APPROXIMATELY 15.0 MILLIGRAMS CHOLESTEROL PER SERVING

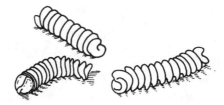

◆ ◆ ◆ ◆ ◆

PENNE IN CREAMY MUSHROOM
SAUCE
(Adapted from Josephine DiDonato)

▶ ▶

Penne is a short, tubular pasta cut on the diagonal and resembling a quill. My friend Josephine invented this recipe and advised, "If you can't find penne, use mezzani, ziti, rigatoni, fusilli, rotelle, even regular spaghetti in a pinch. The thing that matters most is that you choose a pasta of substance, one that will stand up to a cream sauce like this. The pasta should have brass," she went on. "Use nothing delicate or it will be overwhelmed."

This sauce rings so true and is so rich-tasting and altogether luxurious, it's hard to believe it's not laced with heavy cream.

2	teaspoons olive oil
2	large shallots, finely minced
1	medium clove garlic, minced
3/4	pound white mushrooms, wiped clean, trimmed, and thickly sliced
1/4	teaspoon salt, or to taste
3/4	pound penne
1	tablespoon all-purpose flour
1/2	cup low sodium chicken broth
1/4	cup nonfat dry milk
	Freshly ground pepper to taste
2	tablespoons chopped fresh parsley
4	teaspoons freshly grated Parmesan cheese

1. Heat oil in a large nonstick skillet. Add shallots and garlic and sauté over medium-low heat, stirring often, for about 2 minutes or until shallots are wilted. Do not allow shallots and garlic to brown.

2. Add mushrooms and sprinkle with salt, if desired. Raise heat to medium and simmer gently, stirring often, until mushrooms give up their liquid.

3. While mushrooms simmer, slide pasta into boiling water.

4. Sprinkle flour over mushrooms and stir to blend. Reduce heat to medium-low and pour in broth, stirring constantly, until well blended. Sprinkle with dry milk and continue to stir until thickened.

5. When pasta is cooked al dente, drain well and add to mushrooms and sauce in skillet, along with several grindings of pepper. Toss to coat pasta with sauce. (If your skillet is not large enough to hold everything, transfer ingredients to a heated bowl and toss.)

6. Divide among warmed pasta bowls, sprinkle with fresh parsley and Parmesan cheese, and serve immediately.

SERVES 4

APPROXIMATELY 4.0 MILLIGRAMS CHOLESTEROL PER SERVING

◆◆◆◆◆

SPINACH LINGUINE
WITH WALNUT RICOTTA SAUCE

▶ ▶

W alnuts? Cheese? Sure, why not! By combining small quantities of these luscious but fat-laden ingredients, I end up with a creamy, mouth-watering sauce that doesn't throw nutritional caution to the wind—it only seems that way.

³/₄ *pound spinach linguine*
¹/₄ *cup blanched, skinned, chopped walnuts*
1 *clove garlic, pressed*
¹/₄ *cup plus 1 tablespoon chopped fresh parsley*
¹/₄ *cup low sodium chicken broth*
³/₄ *cup low fat ricotta cheese*
   Salt and freshly ground pepper to taste
2 *tablespoons freshly grated Parmesan cheese*

1. Slide pasta into boiling water.
2. While pasta cooks, combine walnuts, garlic, and ¹/₄ cup of the parsley in a food processor. Process, turning machine on and off and scraping down sides, for 10 seconds or until well mixed. Add broth and process until blended to a smooth paste.
3. Transfer mixture to a bowl and add ricotta, stirring with a wooden spoon until ingredients are thoroughly combined. If mixture is very thick, thin with a little of the hot pasta water. Taste and add salt and pepper, if desired.
4. When pasta is cooked, drain and add to ricotta sauce,

---

stirring quickly. Divide among warmed bowls and top each with ½ tablespoon Parmesan cheese.

SERVES 4
APPROXIMATELY 14.0 MILLIGRAMS CHOLESTEROL PER SERVING

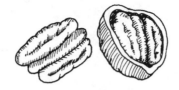

◆ ◆ ◆ ◆

SHELLS WITH TUNA, ARTICHOKES, AND RED PEPPERS

► ►

This is my kind of tuna-helper: a one-dish meal that's colorful, nutritious, and tasty.

3/4   *pound medium shell pasta*
1   *tablespoon olive oil*
2   *cloves garlic, chopped*
1   *small red onion, chopped*
1   *large red bell pepper, seeded and thinly sliced*
1/4   *teaspoon hot red pepper flakes, or to taste*
1/2   *cup dry white wine*
1/2   *cup low sodium chicken broth*
1   *6-ounce jar artichoke hearts, drained and quartered*
10   *black olives, preferably Gaeta, pitted and halved*
1   *6¹/₈-ounce can water-packed light tuna, drained and flaked*
1/4   *cup chopped fresh basil*
   Salt and freshly ground pepper to taste

1. Slide pasta into boiling water.

2. While pasta cooks, heat oil in a nonstick skillet and sauté garlic, onion, and bell pepper over medium-low heat until onion and pepper begin to wilt. Sprinkle with hot pepper flakes if desired, and cook, stirring, for 1 minute.

3. Raise heat to high, add wine and broth, and bring to a boil. Boil for 3 minutes or until liquid is slightly reduced.

Reduce heat to medium and stir in artichoke hearts, olives, and tuna.

4. When pasta is cooked al dente, drain and add to skillet along with basil and salt and pepper, if desired. Toss lightly, divide among warmed pasta bowls, and serve immediately.

SERVES 4

APPROXIMATELY 13.0 MILLIGRAMS CHOLESTEROL PER SERVING

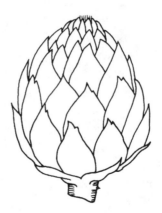

◆◆◆◆◆

SEAFOOD AND PEPPERONCINI LINGUINE

► ►

Not to be confused with pepperoni, that highly seasoned Italian salami, pepperoncini are longish and slender pale green peppers that come to the market either fresh (if you can find them) or conveniently packed in glass jars. Deceptively innocent looking, pepperoncini do have a pleasing kick.

Pimiento strips and coarsely-chopped pepperoncini will lend some dazzle to this dish of linguini with steamed clams and scallops delicately poached in wine, broth, and onions.

1	tablespoon olive oil
3/4	cup dry white wine
20	littleneck clams, scrubbed
3/4	pound linguine
1	small onion, chopped
1/2	cup low sodium chicken broth
1/2	pound sea scallops, rinsed and cut in half if very large
4	large pepperoncini, stemmed, seeded, and coarsely chopped (well-rinsed if packed in brine)
16	pimiento slivers
	Freshly ground black pepper to taste

1. Set pasta water on to boil. At the same time, heat 1/2 tablespoon oil and 1/2 cup of the white wine in a deep skillet large enough to hold all the clams. Add clams, cover tightly,

and steam, shaking pan frequently, for 5 to 6 minutes or until clams have opened. Remove clams with tongs as they open, and set aside (discard any clams that have not opened). Remove skillet from heat, pour off and reserve cooking liquid. Strain liquid, if desired.

2. Slide linguine into boiling water.

3. Return skillet to medium-low heat and add remaining oil. When oil is hot, add onion and sauté, stirring often, until wilted. Do not allow onion to brown.

4. Raise heat to medium-high, add remaining ¼ cup wine and the broth, and simmer until liquid is slightly reduced.

5. Add scallops, reduce heat, and simmer for about 3 minutes or until scallops are nearly white. Return clams and reserved cooking liquid to skillet and just heat through.

6. Drain pasta and add to skillet, tossing to coat well. Divide pasta and seafood among heated bowls, sprinkle each portion with an equal amount of pepperoncini and pimiento strips and a grinding of pepper, and serve immediately.

SERVES 4

APPROXIMATELY 34.0 MILLIGRAMS CHOLESTEROL PER SERVING

♦ ♦ ♦ ♦ ♦

PASTA WITH VODKA

▶ ▶

I find that a pasta of substance, such as fusilli, rigatoni, or penne, is a worthy partner for this lively, robust sauce. The hot pepper and vodka combination provides just the right amount of excitement.

    1   *tablespoon unsalted margarine*
    1   *medium shallot, minced*
  ¹/₄   *cup chopped white onion*
    1   *28-ounce can no-salt-added plum tomatoes,*
        drained and chopped
  ¹/₂   *teaspoon hot pepper flakes, or to taste*
    2   *tablespoons dry red wine*
        Salt to taste
  ³/₄   *pound pasta*
  ¹/₃   *cup evaporated skim milk*
 1¹/₂   *fluid ounces vodka*
  ¹/₄   *cup freshly grated Parmesan cheese*
        Freshly ground pepper to taste

1. Melt margarine in a large, deep, nonstick skillet and sauté shallot and onion over medium-low heat until soft. Do not brown.

2. Raise heat and add tomatoes all at once, then stir in hot pepper flakes, wine, and salt if desired. Meanwhile, slide pasta into boiling water.

3. Bring tomato mixture to a boil, reduce heat, and simmer while the pasta cooks.

4. Drain pasta and add to the pot with the tomatoes,

pour in the evaporated milk and vodka, and sprinkle with the cheese. Heat through over very low flame, stirring, and transfer to warmed plates. Top each plate with a few grindings of pepper.

4 SERVINGS
APPROXIMATELY 5.0 MILLIGRAMS CHOLESTEROL PER SERVING

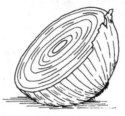

◆◆◆◆◆

PASTA AND ASPARAGUS SALAD
WITH BALSAMIC VINAIGRETTE

▶ ▶

Fresh asparagus is preferred for this dish. If it's unavailable, you can substitute frozen asparagus. But avoid the canned variety, which is too mushy and frequently contains excessive amounts of sodium.

To serve, transfer the completed salad to a platter and bring to the table at room temperature, not chilled.

³/₄	*pound small pasta shells or elbow macaroni*
2	*tablespoons olive oil*
1	*pound fresh asparagus*
2	*cloves garlic, pressed*
6	*scallions, white and tender greens, thinly sliced*
¹/₂	*cup dry white wine*
2	*tablespoons low sodium chicken broth*
3	*tablespoons balsamic vinegar*
1	*tablespoon fresh lemon juice*
	Salt and freshly ground pepper to taste
2	*tablespoons minced fresh basil or parsley*
¹/₄	*cup drained, sliced pimientos*
2	*tablespoons grated Parmesan or Romano cheese*

1. Cook pasta, drain, toss with ¹/₂ tablespoon olive oil, and set aside to cool.

2. While pasta cooks, break off tough ends of asparagus stalks and discard. Rinse asparagus, cut diagonally into 1-inch lengths, and set aside.

3. Heat ½ tablespoon oil in a nonstick skillet. Add asparagus and garlic and cook over medium heat, stirring often, for 3 minutes. Add scallions and wine and bring to a boil. Cover, reduce heat, and simmer gently for 3 minutes or until asparagus is just tender. Remove from heat and let cool.

4. To prepare vinaigrette, combine remaining tablespoon oil with the broth, vinegar, lemon juice, and salt and pepper. Whisk until well blended.

5. When pasta and asparagus mixtures have cooled to room temperature, transfer to a mixing bowl. Add vinaigrette, basil or parsley, and pimientos, and toss until ingredients are thoroughly combined. Sprinkle with grated cheese before serving.

SERVES 4

APPROXIMATELY 2.0 MILLIGRAMS CHOLESTEROL PER SERVING

◆ ◆ ◆ ◆ ◆

WILD RICE
WITH TIPSY CURRANTS

▶ ▶

Imagine the nutlike flavor of wild rice combined with sweet caramelized onions and black currants plumped with wine, then joined by the light, delicate flavor of toasted pine nuts. It's just a hint at the amalgam of textures, colors, and flavors that will confront the palate, then satisfy the soul.

Wonderful with roasts, this dish is equally comfortable with all manner of fowl.

$^1/_2$ cup dried black currants
      Dry white wine
1   cup uncooked wild rice, rinsed
3   cups water
$^1/_3$ cup pine nuts
1   tablespoon olive oil
1   cup coarsely chopped red onion
$^1/_2$ cup low sodium chicken broth
      Salt and freshly ground pepper to taste

1. Sprinkle currants into a small saucepan and pour in enough white wine to cover them by about 1 inch. Heat until wine begins to simmer, then remove saucepan from heat and let currants stand in wine.

2. Combine rice and water in a heavy saucepan and bring to a boil. Reduce heat, cover, and simmer gently for about 50 minutes or until rice is tender and grains begin to split.

3. While rice cooks, scatter pine nuts into a nonstick skillet in one layer and heat over a low flame, shaking pan frequently, until nuts are lightly golden. Transfer to a small bowl and let cool.

4. When rice is nearly cooked, heat oil in skillet and sauté onion over medium heat, stirring occasionally, until translucent. Raise heat to medium-high, add broth, and cook for 2 minutes.

5. When rice is cooked, pour off any remaining liquid, fluff with a fork, and transfer rice to skillet.

6. Drain currants, reserving 2 tablespoons of the wine. Add reserved wine to rice in skillet, along with currants, pine nuts, and salt and pepper to taste. Toss to combine ingredients and serve.

SERVES 4

APPROXIMATELY .5 MILLIGRAM CHOLESTEROL PER SERVING

TURMERIC RICE

◆ ◆

Turmeric is the root of a tropical plant that imparts a pungent flavor and a yellowish-orange cast. Almost always used in curry preparations, turmeric is also a major ingredient in mustard, lending its flavor and bright yellow color to both products.

Turmeric Rice is the logical accompaniment for Tandoori Chicken (page 77) or with simply baked or roasted poultry.

1	tablespoon unsalted margarine
1	large shallot, minced, or 2 tablespoons finely chopped onion
1	cup uncooked long-grain white rice
2	cups low sodium chicken broth
	Juice of 1 large lemon
$^1/_2$	teaspoon turmeric
$^1/_4$	teaspoon ground coriander
$^1/_4$	cup chopped fresh cilantro or parsley
$^1/_4$	cup golden raisins (optional)

1. Heat margarine in a medium nonstick pot and sauté shallot or onion, stirring frequently, until wilted but not browned. Add rice and cook, stirring with a wooden spoon, until rice begins to color.

2. Raise heat, add broth, lemon juice, turmeric, and coriander, and bring to a boil. Cover, reduce heat, and simmer gently for about 25 minutes or until rice is just tender.

3. Remove from heat, stir in cilantro and raisins if desired. Cover and let sit for 5 minutes before serving.

SERVES 4
APPROXIMATELY 3.0 MILLIGRAMS CHOLESTEROL PER SERVING

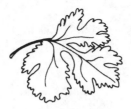

♦♦♦♦♦

BROWN RICE
AND CONFETTI VEGETABLES

▶▶▶▶▶▶▶▶▶▶▶▶▶▶▶▶▶▶▶▶▶▶▶

$\mathbb{A}$s festive as confetti on New Year's Eve, this colorful dish is perfect at any time of the year. Tasty, texturally interesting, and packed with good nutrition, it makes a wonderful component of well-planned vegetarian dinners.

2¹/₂	cups water (lightly salted, if desired)
1	cup uncooked brown rice
1¹/₂	tablespoons canola or other light oil
1	clove garlic, finely minced
1	small onion, finely diced
1	carrot, finely diced
1	stalk celery, finely diced
¹/₂	green or red bell pepper, finely diced
¹/₂	cup corn kernels, fresh, or frozen and thawed
2	ripe plum tomatoes, chopped
¹/₂	cup low sodium tomato sauce
2	tablespoons fresh lemon juice
2	tablespoons minced fresh cilantro or parsley
	Salt and freshly ground pepper to taste

1. Bring water to a boil, add rice, cover, reduce heat, and simmer for 45 minutes or until rice is just tender. Remove from heat, drain off any excess liquid, and let stand covered to keep warm.

2. Heat oil in a large nonstick skillet. Add garlic, onion,

---

carrot, celery, bell pepper, and corn. Cook over medium-low heat, stirring often, for 5 minutes. Add tomatoes and cook for an additional 2 minutes.

    3. Add tomato sauce, lemon juice, cilantro or parsley, and salt and pepper to taste. Stir for 1 minute or until ingredients are well blended. Stir in rice and heat through. Serve immediately.

SERVES 4

0 MILLIGRAMS CHOLESTEROL PER RECIPE

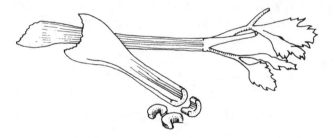

◆◆◆◆◆

BARLEY AND MUSHROOM CASSEROLE

▶ ▶

Serve this savory dish as a change of pace from rice and the usual bread-based stuffings. Excellent alongside poultry, it also goes well with roasted meats and steamed or grilled fish (such as bluefish, swordfish, or salmon) or as part of a vegetarian meal (substitute vegetable broth for the beef broth used in the recipe below).

2	teaspoons olive or vegetable oil
1	medium onion, coarsely chopped
¹/₂	pound firm white mushrooms, wiped clean and sliced
	Dash hot pepper sauce, or to taste
1	cup uncooked pearled barley
¹/₄	teaspoon dried summer savory
¹/₄	teaspoon dried rosemary
¹/₄	teaspoon dried thyme
	Vegetable oil cooking spray
2	cups low sodium beef broth
¹/₄	cup chopped fresh parsley
¹/₄	cup fresh lemon juice
	Salt and freshly ground pepper to taste

1. Preheat oven to 350°F.

2. Heat oil in nonstick skillet and sauté onion and mushrooms over medium-low heat until onion is well wilted and mushrooms have given up their liquid. Swirl in a dash of hot pepper sauce if desired.

---

3. Add barley and herbs and shake skillet over medium heat for about 1 minute or until barley is coated with onion mixture.

4. Transfer contents of skillet to an ovenproof casserole lightly coated with cooking spray. Pour in 1 cup of broth, cover, and bake for 20 minutes. Add second cup of broth, cover, and return to oven for another 25 minutes or until liquid has been absorbed.

5. Remove cover, sprinkle with parsley and lemon juice, and toss well with a fork. Taste, add salt and pepper if desired, and serve very hot.

SERVES 4

APPROXIMATELY .5 MILLIGRAM CHOLESTEROL PER SERVING

◆ ◆ ◆ ◆ ◆

BASIC POLENTA

▶ ▶

If you don't care to use any of the instant polenta mixes available, this traditional method is time consuming but rewarding in both flavor and consistency.

6³/₄ *cups water*
¹/₂ *teaspoon salt, or to taste*
1³/₄ *cups yellow cornmeal (preferably coarse or medium grain)*
¹/₄ *teaspoon each dried thyme and rosemary (optional)*
Vegetable oil cooking spray

1. Combine water and salt in a large saucepan and bring to a boil. Gradually add cornmeal to boiling water, stirring constantly. When all of the cornmeal has been incorporated, add herbs, reduce heat, and cook at the barest simmer, stirring often, for about 35 minutes or until the polenta is thick and creamy.

2. Lightly coat an 8-inch-square baking pan with cooking spray and pour in the cooked polenta. Set aside to cool. When completely cool, polenta can be cut in squares, grilled, or baked in a recipe.

MAKES 6 SQUARES
0 MILLIGRAMS CHOLESTEROL PER RECIPE

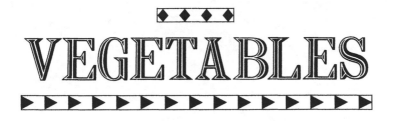

VEGETABLES

◆ ◆ ◆ ◆ ◆

PAN-ROASTED ARTICHOKE HEARTS, ONIONS, AND POTATOES

▶ ▶

Easy to execute but hard to resist, this wonderful combination is a side dish that goes well with almost anything.

    1   16-ounce can water-packed artichoke hearts,
        drained
   12   small white boiling onions, peeled
    1   bay leaf
   ½   teaspoon dried thyme
   ½   teaspoon dried summer savory
    1   large clove garlic, quartered
   12   tiny new potatoes, carefully peeled to retain shape
    1   cup low sodium chicken broth
        Salt and freshly ground pepper to taste
        Juice of 1 large lemon

1. In a deep skillet, combine all ingredients, except salt, pepper, and lemon juice. Cover and cook over medium-low heat for 30 minutes or until potatoes are tender and liquid is nearly absorbed. Raise heat and cook briefly, uncovered, until potatoes and artichokes are golden in spots.

2. Remove bay leaf and transfer vegetables to a heated platter. Sprinkle with salt, pepper, and lemon juice and serve hot.

SERVES 4
APPROXIMATELY 1.0 MILLIGRAM CHOLESTEROL PER SERVING

◆◆◆◆◆

BROCCOLI WITH LEMON
MUSTARD SAUCE

▶▶▶▶▶▶▶▶▶▶▶▶▶▶▶▶▶▶▶▶▶▶▶▶

I think most people interested in nutrition have by now heard about studies indicating that broccoli is one of the possible anticancer vegetables. It's so highly doctor-recommended that a United States president complained he was being served entirely too much of it.

Yes, steamed broccoli is good nourishment. And with this savory lemon mustard sauce, it's tasty eating too.

> 1   *large head broccoli*
> 2   *teaspoons sugar*
> 2   *teaspoons white wine vinegar*
> 1   *teaspoon cornstarch*
> ¹/₄ *cup cold water*
> ¹/₄ *cup low sodium chicken broth*
> 3   *tablespoons fresh lemon juice*
> 1   *tablespoon Dijon mustard*
> ¹/₂ *teaspoon Worcestershire sauce*
>   *Salt to taste*

1. Trim broccoli, discarding tough bottom stems, rinse, and quarter or separate into florets. Steam broccoli until just tender.

2. While broccoli steams, prepare sauce by combining sugar and vinegar in a small saucepan. Bring to a boil, reduce heat, and cook, stirring often, for about 3 minutes or until sugar is dissolved and mixture begins to color.

3. Dissolve cornstarch in cold water and add to sauce-

---

pan. Stir in broth, lemon juice, mustard, and Worcestershire. Bring mixture to a boil and cook, stirring constantly, for 2 minutes or until ingredients are well blended. Taste and add salt, if desired.

4. Transfer steamed broccoli to a warm platter, top with sauce, and serve.

SERVES 4

APPROXIMATELY .3 MILLIGRAM CHOLESTEROL PER SERVING

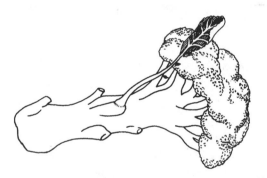

◆ ◆ ◆ ◆ ◆

CREAMY MASHED POTATOES
WITH SCALLIONS

▶ ▶

It's possible to enjoy a large helping of smooth, creamy mashed potatoes without being concerned about how much cholesterol it contains. My adaptation has the taste of real-cream mashed potatoes, plus the added flavor of scallions.

For a spectacular presentation, pipe the potatoes through a pastry bag fitted with a star tip and run briefly under the broiler.

4   *medium baking potatoes, peeled and cubed*
2   *tablespoons unsalted margarine*
6   *scallions, white and tender greens, finely sliced*
1   *tablespoon minced fresh parsley or ¹/₂ tablespoon dried*
1   *cup evaporated skim milk*
    Salt and freshly ground pepper to taste

1. Boil potatoes in water (lightly salted, if desired) for about 20 minutes or until tender.

2. While potatoes cook, heat margarine in a small skillet and sauté scallions over medium heat until lightly browned.

3. When potatoes are done, remove from heat and drain well. Return potatoes to pot and cook briefly over low heat, shaking pot, to evaporate any remaining moisture.

4. Add scallions and margarine to potatoes along with remaining ingredients and mash until smooth and well

blended. Serve immediately or transfer to a baking dish and keep warm in the oven until ready to serve.

SERVES 4
APPROXIMATELY 2.5 MILLIGRAMS CHOLESTEROL PER SERVING

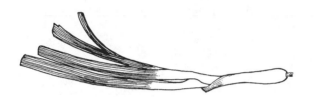

♦ ♦ ♦ ♦ ♦

TWICE-BAKED POTATOES

▶ ▶

Potatoes that are baked, mashed, returned to their shells, and baked again are delicious. And this recipe—where the potatoes are mashed with shallots, a touch of garlic, parsley, and olive oil, instead of the usual butter and milk—is one of the best! Try it with sweet potatoes too.

> 2 *large baking potatoes*
> 2 *shallots, finely minced*
> 1 *small clove garlic, finely minced*
> 1 *tablespoon chopped fresh parsley or* $^{1}/_{2}$ *tablespoon dried*
> 2 *tablespoons olive oil*
>   *Salt and freshly ground pepper to taste*

1. Preheat oven to 350°F.

2. Wash potatoes and pierce skins with a fork. Bake for about 45 minutes or until just tender. Remove potatoes from oven, but do not turn off heat.

3. Cut potatoes in half lengthwise. Keeping skins intact, carefully scoop out pulp and transfer to a mixing bowl; reserve skins.

4. Mash pulp with remaining ingredients and divide mixture evenly among potato skins. Return to oven and bake for 15 minutes.

SERVES 4

0 MILLIGRAMS CHOLESTEROL PER RECIPE

◆◆◆◆◆

SAUTÉED CHERRY TOMATOES

▶▶▶▶▶▶▶▶▶▶▶▶▶▶▶▶▶▶▶▶▶▶▶▶▶

Bursting with the vibrant colors and flavors reminiscent of Provence, this herb-scented tomato, garlic, and black olive combination will enhance any simply prepared meat, poultry, or fish entrée. (I confess I sometimes just spoon this voluptuous blend on good, crusty French bread or lavish a steamed piece of fish with it.)

12	*large cherry tomatoes (1½-inch diameter) or 8 small regular tomatoes (2-inch diameter)*
1	*teaspoon olive oil*
1	*clove garlic, peeled and flattened*
½	*cup low sodium chicken broth*
1	*teaspoon chopped fresh thyme or ½ teaspoon dried*
	Pinch sugar
10	*large black olives, pitted and halved*
1	*tablespoon chopped fresh basil*
	Salt and freshly ground pepper to taste

1. Drop tomatoes, a few at a time, into boiling water for 30 seconds. Remove and plunge quickly into cold water. Peel tomatoes carefully and set aside. Repeat until all tomatoes have been peeled.

2. Heat oil in a deep nonstick skillet large enough to hold all tomatoes in one layer. Sauté garlic over medium-low heat until soft, stirring occasionally. Do not brown.

3. Raise heat and add broth. Cook for 1 minute, then

reduce heat to medium-low and carefully add tomatoes. Sprinkle with thyme and sugar and add olive halves.

4. Cover and simmer gently for about 10 minutes or until tomatoes are tender but still retain shape. Serve sprinkled with basil and salt and pepper, if desired.

SERVES 4

APPROXIMATELY .5 MILLIGRAM CHOLESTEROL PER SERVING

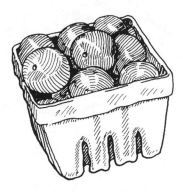

◆ ◆ ◆ ◆ ◆

SPANISH ONIONS STUFFED
WITH CHICKEN AND MUSHROOMS

▶ ▶

Sort of an onion surprise, this dish makes a light yet splendid meal.

4   *medium Spanish onions, peeled*
1   *small stalk celery, cut in half*
1   *small onion, quartered*
¹/₂   *boneless, skinless chicken breast (about ¹/₄ pound)*
¹/₂   *cup chopped fresh mushrooms*
¹/₂   *cup coarse bread crumbs, preferably made from day-old French bread*
¹/₄   *teaspoon each: dried thyme, rosemary, tarragon, or your favorite herb mixture*
      Salt and freshly ground pepper to taste
2   *tablespoons low sodium chicken broth*
1   *tablespoon dry sherry*
      Water or dry white wine
      Paprika (optional)

1. In a large saucepan, cover Spanish onions with water, bring to a boil, adjust heat, and simmer for 15 minutes or until onions are nearly tender but not mushy or limp. Remove onions from water with slotted spoon and let cool. Reserve 1 cup of the water.

2. To reserved water, add celery and quartered onion, bring to a boil, and cook 5 minutes. Add chicken, cover, reduce heat, and cook at a bare simmer for 15 minutes.

Remove saucepan from heat but leave covered and allow chicken to cool in the liquid.

3. When Spanish onions have cooled, cut ⅓ inch off tops and carefully scoop out onion pulp with the small end of a melon baller or a grapefruit spoon, leaving a ½-inch shell. Reserve pulp from 1 onion. Invert onion shells and drain.

4. Preheat oven to 375°F.

5. When chicken has cooled to room temperature, remove chicken and celery from poaching liquid. Cut chicken into tiny cubes or shred coarsely and transfer to a mixing bowl. Chop reserved onion pulp and celery and add to bowl, along with mushrooms, bread crumbs, herbs, salt if desired, and generous grindings of pepper. Moisten mixture with broth and sherry, and toss with a fork until ingredients are thoroughly blended.

6. Stuff onion cavities with chicken mixture. Place stuffed onions upright in a small baking dish. Pour in water or wine to a depth of no more than ¼ inch. Bake, uncovered, for about 45 minutes or until tender and lightly golden. If onions begin to brown within the first half hour of cooking, tent loosely with foil for the final 15 minutes. Sprinkle lightly with paprika before serving, if desired.

SERVES 4

APPROXIMATELY 16.0 MILLIGRAMS CHOLESTEROL PER SERVING

◆ ◆ ◆ ◆ ◆

BUTTERNUT SQUASH
WITH BROWN SUGAR GLAZE

▶ ▶

A painless way of pulling ourselves up and out of the sweet potato pie rut we sometimes find ourselves sinking into Thanksgiving after Thanksgiving, Christmas after Easter after Rosh Hashanah, et cetera, is with this delightful casserole of butternut squash.

6   cups peeled, cubed fresh butternut squash
3   tablespoons low fat (1%) milk
2   tablespoons light brown sugar
1   teaspoon freshly grated ginger root or ¹/₂ teaspoon powdered
    Freshly ground pepper to taste
1   tablespoon honey
¹/₄ cup chopped walnuts (optional)

1. Cook squash in boiling water (lightly salted, if desired) until tender. Drain well and transfer to a mixing bowl.

2. Preheat oven to 350°F.

3. Mash squash together with milk, 1 tablespoon brown sugar, ginger, and freshly ground pepper. Spread mixture into an ovenproof casserole. Sprinkle top with remaining brown sugar, drizzle with honey, and sprinkle with walnuts if desired.

4. Bake for 20 minutes. Serve immediately.

SERVES 4

APPROXIMATELY .5 MILLIGRAM CHOLESTEROL PER SERVING

◆ ◆ ◆ ◆ ◆

LEEK AND POTATO PIE

▶ ▶

Resembling scallions with thyroid conditions, leeks are nonetheless the crowned heads of the onion family. Essential to the success of many basic stocks, stews, and sauces, leeks are also partners in crime in creating that artery mugger, vichyssoise—the very elegant French leek and potato soup. (See my Light Vichyssoise, page 51.)

This recipe rounds up the usual suspects—the leek and potato gang—this time disarming them as the enemy and casting them instead in a more satisfactory role: friendly, soothing. Serve as a first course, hors d'oeuvre, light lunch, or dinner entrée, perhaps with just a salad of mixed greens.

　　　Vegetable oil cooking spray
1　tablespoon olive oil
2　medium leeks, white and tender greens, rinsed
　　　and chopped
1　tablespoon flour
¼　cup low sodium chicken broth
2　tablespoons nonfat dry milk
2　large egg whites, lightly beaten
　　　Salt and freshly ground pepper to taste
4　medium potatoes, peeled and sliced
1　cup evaporated skim milk

1. Coat an 8-inch-square baking dish lightly with cooking spray and set aside.

2. Heat oil in a nonstick skillet and sauté leeks over

medium-low heat until softened. Add flour and stir to dissolve. Pour in broth, sprinkle with nonfat dry milk, and continue to cook, stirring constantly, until mixture is creamy and thickened slightly. Remove from heat and whisk in egg whites and salt and pepper. Meanwhile, preheat oven to 375°F.

3. In the prepared baking dish, alternate rows of potato slices and leek mixture, ending with leeks. Pour evaporated milk over all. Bake for 40 minutes or until set. Cut into squares and serve.

SERVES 6

APPROXIMATELY 2.0 MILLIGRAMS CHOLESTEROL PER SERVING

♦♦♦♦♦

CORN "OYSTERS"

▶▶▶▶▶▶▶▶▶▶▶▶▶▶▶▶▶▶▶▶▶▶▶▶▶

§omehow, these terrific "oysters" always find their way back to the bed . . . my bed, that is. Because I love to nibble on these savory corn critters with a little maple syrup on the side as my breakfast, brunch, or luncheon in bed. They are equally good alongside grilled or barbecued chicken or turkey and a steamed vegetable or slaw.

 1 *cup corn kernels, fresh, or frozen and thawed*
 3 *tablespoons drained, diced pimientos*
 2 *egg whites*
 ¹/₄ *cup all-purpose flour*
 ¹/₂ *teaspoon baking powder*
   Salt and freshly ground pepper to taste
   Vegetable oil cooking spray
 1 *tablespoon peanut oil*
   Maple syrup (optional)

1. In a mixing bowl, combine corn and pimientos with egg whites and stir lightly to blend. Add flour, baking powder, and salt and pepper to taste. Mix until ingredients are thoroughly blended.

2. Heat peanut oil in a large nonstick skillet coated with cooking spray. Drop "oysters" by the tablespoonful into skillet, being careful that they do not touch each other (if necessary, do this in two or three batches). Cook over medium heat until golden, then turn and brown the other side. Remove to

a heated platter and keep warm. Serve hot with maple syrup if desired.

MAKES ABOUT 8 "OYSTERS"
0 MILLIGRAMS CHOLESTEROL PER RECIPE

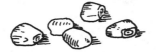

◆◆◆◆◆

CREAMED SPINACH

▶▶▶▶▶▶▶▶▶▶▶▶▶▶▶▶▶▶▶▶▶▶▶▶

Here's a low-freight version of one of my all-time favorite recipes. As a side dish it's great with just about any grilled, poached, baked, or sautéed fish, meat, or fowl. It also makes a terrific filling for baked potatoes, or a bed or topping for steamed fish.

1½ pounds fresh spinach, trimmed, rinsed, and drained
1 tablespoon unsalted margarine
1 tablespoon flour
½ cup evaporated skim milk
Salt and freshly ground pepper to taste
¼ teaspoon ground nutmeg, or to taste

1. Steam spinach until well wilted, then transfer to a colander to drain. When cool enough to handle, press to squeeze out excess moisture.
2. Melt margarine in a skillet over medium heat. Remove from heat, add flour, and stir until smooth. Return to heat and slowly add milk, stirring constantly, until mixture just starts to simmer. Remove from heat and season to taste with salt, pepper, and nutmeg if desired.
3. Chop spinach, add to skillet, and cook over very low heat, stirring constantly, for 1 minute or until heated through.

SERVES 4

APPROXIMATELY 1.0 MILLIGRAM CHOLESTEROL PER SERVING

◆◆◆◆◆

CREAMED ONIONS WITH THYME

▶▶▶▶▶▶▶▶▶▶▶▶▶▶▶▶▶▶▶▶▶▶▶▶▶▶

Don't reserve this stunning dish for your holiday table. Serve it with any simple roast or try it with my Apple-Glazed Chicken (page 87) or Mushroom-Stuffed Turkey in Wine Sauce (page 97).

> 1   *pound small white boiling onions*
> 1¹/₂ *cups low sodium chicken broth*
> 1   *bay leaf*
> 1   *cup Medium White Sauce (page 11)*
> 1¹/₂ *teaspoons chopped fresh thyme or ¹/₂ teaspoon*
>   *dried*
>   *Pinch nutmeg*
>   *Salt and white pepper to taste*

1. Drop onions into a pot of boiling water and boil for 1 minute. Drain and set aside to cool slightly. When just cool enough to handle, slip off skins, lightly trim stem and root ends, and cut a small slash in the root end.

2. In a saucepan, combine onions with broth and bay leaf, cover, and bring to a simmer. Cook over medium-low heat for 30 minutes or until onions are tender but still whole.

3. In a small mixing bowl, combine Medium White Sauce with thyme, nutmeg, and salt and pepper to taste.

4. When onions are tender, drain, remove bay leaf, and reserve ¹/₂ cup of cooking liquid. Return onions to saucepan, add ¹/₄ cup of the reserved liquid and the cream sauce. Stir over very low heat until heated through and well blended.

Add additional broth by the spoonful if sauce is too thick. Taste and add additional seasonings, if desired. Serve at once.

SERVES 4
APPROXIMATELY 4.0 MILLIGRAMS CHOLESTEROL PER SERVING

♦ ♦ ♦ ♦

CARROT SLAW
WITH CREAMY MINT DRESSING

▶ ▶

$\mathbb{D}$elightful on the lips and kind to the hips, this slaw is one of the stalwarts of summer. Great with broiled chicken, to take along on a picnic, on the terrace or patio, as a first course, or to augment any light meal.

> 3 *medium carrots*
> 1 *tablespoon fresh lemon juice*
> ¹/₂ *red onion, finely minced*
> ¹/₂ *cup Mock Mayonnaise (page 4)*
>   *Salt and freshly ground pepper to taste*
> 1 *tablespoon minced fresh mint or ¹/₂ tablespoon dried*

1. Shred or grate carrots coarsely, using a vegetable parer, food processor, or hand grater. Transfer to a mixing bowl and toss with lemon juice and onion.

2. Whisk together Mock Mayonnaise, salt and pepper to taste, and mint. Add to carrots in bowl and toss until ingredients are well blended. Cover and chill for about 1 hour before serving.

SERVES 4

APPROXIMATELY 2.0 MILLIGRAMS CHOLESTEROL PER SERVING

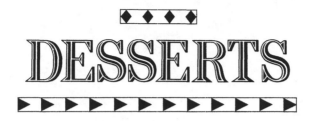

DESSERTS

◆◆◆◆◆

ORANGE ANGEL FOOD CAKE

▶▶▶▶▶▶▶▶▶▶▶▶▶▶▶▶▶▶▶▶▶▶▶▶▶▶

With zero cholesterol, angel food cake is almost an imperative for the dessert lover on a strict low cholesterol regime. However, most angel food desserts are heavily laden with sugar. I prefer to substitute a fruit extract for some of the sugar, as I've done here, or to garnish my plate with a naturally sweetened fruit sauce.

To assure optimal results, sift the flour several times and be sure to use grease-free utensils.

1	cup cake flour, sifted
1/4	teaspoon salt
3/4	cup sugar
10	large egg whites, at room temperature
3/4	teaspoon cream of tartar
2	tablespoons fresh orange juice
1 1/2	teaspoons orange extract
1	tablespoon grated orange zest

1. Preheat oven to 325°F. Position rack in lower third of oven.

2. Resift flour together with salt and 1/2 cup sugar.

3. In a grease-free nonaluminum bowl, combine egg whites with cream of tartar and beat until frothy. Gradually add remaining 1/4 cup sugar and continue to beat egg whites until soft peaks form. Add orange juice, extract, and zest, and beat until egg whites are stiff but not dry.

4. Sift the flour mixture over the egg whites in three batches and fold in gently but quickly after each addition.

---

5. Pour batter into a clean, *ungreased* 10-inch tube pan. Run a very clean knife through the batter once to eliminate air bubbles. Bake for about 50 minutes or until a tester inserted in the center comes out clean. Cake will pull away from the sides of the pan when it is done.

6. Invert pan onto a funnel turned upside down (the hole in the tube pan should fit over the point of the funnel) and cool cake thoroughly in pan.

SERVES 12

0 MILLIGRAMS CHOLESTEROL PER RECIPE

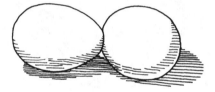

◆◆◆◆◆

MOCHA CHOCOLATE CHIP MERINGUES

▶▶▶▶▶▶▶▶▶▶▶▶▶▶▶▶▶▶▶▶▶▶▶▶

These delightfully light meringues are easy to make, deliciously chewy, and full of coffee-chocolatey flavor.

1 *ounce semisweet chocolate, finely chopped or ground*
4 *tablespoons cocoa powder*
1 *tablespoon flour*
¼ *teaspoon ground cinnamon*
1 *tablespoon instant espresso powder*
4 *large egg whites, at room temperature*
⅛ *teaspoon cream of tartar*
3 *tablespoons confectioners' sugar*
¼ *cup mini chocolate chips*

1. Preheat oven to 250°F. Line the surface of 2 large cookie sheets with baking parchment.

2. In a small bowl, combine the chocolate, cocoa, flour, cinnamon, and espresso powder, sifting if necessary to eliminate lumps, and set aside.

3. In a large, grease-free bowl, beat egg whites until frothy. Add cream of tartar and beat at high speed until soft peaks form. Add sugar gradually and beat until stiff peaks form.

4. Very gently but quickly fold about half of the cocoa mixture into the egg whites until blended. Repeat with the remaining cocoa mixture, then fold in the chocolate chips.

Drop batter by heaping teaspoonfuls onto the cookie sheets, leaving about 1½ inches between cookies. Bake for about 25 minutes or until just firm on top. Remove from oven and place cookie sheets on a rack. When cool, the cookies should slide off.

MAKES ABOUT 30 COOKIES
0 MILLIGRAMS CHOLESTEROL PER RECIPE

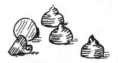

◆ ◆ ◆ ◆ ◆

NO-BAKE CHEESECAKE

▶ ▶

This refreshing lemony cheesecake is really simple to prepare if you have a food processor. Once the ingredients are combined, you need only to chill it and relax.

1	tablespoon light unsalted margarine
¹/₂	cup graham cracker crumbs
2	envelopes unflavored gelatin
¹/₂	cup cold water
1	cup low fat (1%) milk
1	cup low fat (1%) cottage cheese
1	cup low fat ricotta cheese
³/₄	cup sifted sugar
¹/₂	teaspoon vanilla extract
1	tablespoon grated lemon rind
4	tablespoons fresh lemon juice
¹/₈	teaspoon salt

1. Grease the bottom and sides of an 8-inch springform pan with the margarine and sprinkle with graham cracker crumbs. Press crumbs firmly onto sides and bottom of pan. Refrigerate for at least 30 minutes.

2. In the work bowl of a food processor, sprinkle gelatin over cold water and let stand 3 minutes.

3. Meanwhile, heat milk in a small saucepan over low heat to just below simmering. Pour immediately into bowl of the food processor and process for about 10 seconds or until gelatin is completely dissolved.

4. Add remaining ingredients to food processor and puree until smooth and creamy. Pour mixture into prepared springform pan and refrigerate for about 2 hours or until set.

SERVES 8
APPROXIMATELY 12.0 MILLIGRAMS CHOLESTEROL PER SERVING

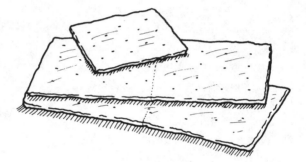

◆◆◆◆◆

SPICED PEACH SOUFFLÉ
WITH FRESH RASPBERRY SAUCE

▶ ▶

Light and airy, redolent of peaches, cinnamon, allspice, and nutmeg, this impressive dessert is a real crowd-pleaser.

The elegant raspberry sauce can also be spooned over poached peaches or pears, lemon sorbet, or frozen yogurt.

 1 *pound fresh ripe peaches or 2 cups canned in juice, juice reserved*
 1 *tablespoon fresh lemon juice if using fresh peaches*
 2 *tablespoons cornstarch*
 ¼ *cup water or peach nectar or reserved peach juice*
 4 *tablespoons sugar*
 1 *teaspoon vanilla extract*
 ¼ *teaspoon each ground cinnamon, allspice, and nutmeg*
    Vegetable oil cooking spray
 5 *large egg whites, at room temperature*
 ¼ *teaspoon cream of tartar*

RASPBERRY SAUCE
 1 *pint fresh raspberries, picked over and rinsed*
 1 *tablespoon fresh lemon juice*
 2 *teaspoons superfine sugar if berries are tart*
 1 *tablespoon cognac or brandy (optional)*

1. If using fresh peaches, blanch them in boiling water for 1 minute, then plunge quickly into cold water. Peel, cut in half, remove pits, slice, and toss with lemon juice.

---

2. Puree peaches in food processor, then transfer to a small saucepan.

3. Dissolve cornstarch in water or nectar and stir into peaches in saucepan. Add 3 tablespoons sugar, vanilla extract, and spices and bring to a boil. Reduce heat to low and cook, stirring often, for about 5 minutes or until smooth and thickened. Transfer mixture to a small bowl and cool until just barely warm. Do not refrigerate.

4. While peach mixture cools, preheat oven to 375°F. Spray a 1-quart soufflé dish with cooking spray and set aside.

5. Beat egg whites until frothy, then sprinkle with cream of tartar and beat until soft peaks form. Sprinkle in remaining sugar and beat until stiff peaks form. Fold the sauce into the whites in three batches, working gently but quickly. Turn the mixture into prepared dish and bake for 30 minutes or until set and very puffy.

6. While soufflé bakes, prepare raspberry sauce: Puree raspberries and strain seeds, if desired. Combine with lemon juice, sugar, and brandy in a saucepan and bring to a boil. If mixture seems dry, add water by the spoonful. Remove from heat and let cool slightly.

7. When soufflé is done, serve immediately with sauce.

SERVES 6

0 MILLIGRAMS CHOLESTEROL PER RECIPE

LEMON CAKE WITH BLUEBERRY SAUCE

▶ ▶

A wonderful addition to a low cholesterol repertoire, this festive dessert is also low in fat and calories. Serve it with the blueberry sauce or with any other fruit or fruit sauce.

	Vegetable oil cooking spray
1	tablespoon plus 1¹/₂ cups sifted cake flour
³/₄	cup plus 1 tablespoon sugar
1	teaspoon baking powder
1	teaspoon baking soda
¹/₄	teaspoon salt
1	tablespoon grated fresh lemon zest
7	large egg whites, at room temperature
¹/₄	teaspoon cream of tartar
¹/₄	cup safflower oil
²/₃	cup warm water
¹/₄	cup fresh lemon juice
1	teaspoon almond extract
	Confectioners' sugar

BLUEBERRY SAUCE

1	cup blueberries, picked over and rinsed
1	tablespoon sugar
1	tablespoon fresh lemon juice

1. Preheat oven to 350°F. Coat a 10-inch Bundt pan with cooking spray and 1 tablespoon flour, tapping out any excess. Set pan aside.

2. Sift together remaining 1½ cups flour, ¾ cup sugar, baking powder and soda, salt, and lemon zest and set aside.

3. In large, grease-free mixing bowl, beat egg whites until frothy. Add cream of tartar and beat until soft peaks form, then add 1 tablespoon sugar and beat until stiff peaks form.

4. Make a well in the center of flour mixture and add oil, water, ¼ cup lemon juice, and almond extract. Mix until just blended.

5. Fold flour mixture into egg whites in three batches, working gently but quickly just to blend.

6. Scrape batter into prepared pan and bake in center of oven for about 45 minutes or until tester inserted in center comes out clean. Cool for 10 minutes on rack, then remove cake from pan and cool completely.

7. While cake cools, prepare blueberry sauce. Combine berries and 1 tablespoon sugar in food processor and puree. Transfer to a small saucepan, add 1 tablespoon lemon juice, and heat to boiling. If mixture is very thick, add a small amount of water to bring to desired consistency. Cool and refrigerate until serving time.

8. To serve, sprinkle cake lightly with confectioners' sugar and serve slices on individual plates of blueberry sauce.

SERVES 12

0 MILLIGRAMS CHOLESTEROL PER RECIPE

◆ ◆ ◆ ◆ ◆

CHOCOLATE ORANGE
CHIFFON CAKE

▶ ▶

I f you wish, you can substitute a different fruit extract for the orange and eliminate the zest, or, for the chocoholics of the crowd, omit the fruit entirely.

	Vegetable oil cooking spray
1¹/₂	*cups sifted cake flour plus extra for preparing pan*
6	*large egg whites, at room temperature*
¹/₄	*teaspoon cream of tartar*
1¹/₄	*cups plus 2 tablespoons sugar*
¹/₃	*cup unsweetened cocoa*
2	*teaspoons baking powder*
¹/₄	*teaspoon salt*
2	*tablespoons grated orange zest*
¹/₂	*cup safflower oil*
²/₃	*cup warm water*
1	*teaspoon vanilla extract*
2	*teaspoons orange extract*

1. Preheat oven to 350°F. Position rack in center of oven. Coat a 10-inch Bundt pan with cooking spray and sprinkle with flour, tapping to shake out excess. Set aside.

2. In large, grease-free mixing bowl, beat egg whites with cream of tartar until soft peaks form. Add 2 tablespoons sugar and beat until stiff but not dry.

3. Sift together flour, cocoa, 1¹/₄ cups sugar, baking powder, and salt. Sprinkle in orange zest. Make a deep well in

the center and add oil, water, and extracts. Mix until just blended.

4. Fold flour mixture into egg whites in three batches, working gently but quickly.

5. Pour batter into prepared pan and bake for 45 minutes or until tester inserted in center of cake comes out clean.

6. Cool 15 minutes on rack. Remove from pan and cool completely.

SERVES 12

0 MILLIGRAMS CHOLESTEROL PER RECIPE

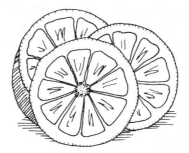

♦ ♦ ♦ ♦ ♦

DANISH BUTTERMILK MOUSSE

▶ ▶

Simple, lovely, deceptively light, and absolutely delicious. Serve sauced with cold, cooked, stewed, or pureed fruit.

> ³/₄ cup evaporated skim milk
> 1 envelope unflavored gelatin
> ¹/₄ cup cold water
> 1 cup low fat buttermilk
> 3 tablespoons sugar
> 1 teaspoon vanilla extract
> 1 teaspoon almond extract
> 1 teaspoon grated lemon zest

1. Pour evaporated milk into a bowl and freeze bowl and beaters for 1 hour or until a large rim of slush forms in the bowl.

2. In the top of a double boiler, sprinkle gelatin over cold water and let sit 2 to 3 minutes. Heat water and stir until gelatin is dissolved.

3. Mix together buttermilk, sugar, extracts, and lemon zest. Fold into gelatin mixture and chill until it just begins to set.

4. Remove chilled milk from freezer and whip until stiff. Fold whipped milk into cooled buttermilk mixture, pour mousse into individual serving dishes, and chill for 1 hour or until completely set.

SERVES 4

APPROXIMATELY 4.0 MILLIGRAMS CHOLESTEROL PER SERVING

◆ ◆ ◆ ◆ ◆

FROZEN CINNAMON YOGURT

▶ ▶

G reat by itself or scooped over slices of warmed apple pie. This recipe is easily doubled and keeps well, tightly covered, in the freezer.

16   *ounces low fat vanilla yogurt*
1   *teaspoon ground cinnamon*
1/2   *teaspoon vanilla extract*

1. Combine all ingredients and whisk to blend well. Spread mixture into shallow trays and freeze until slushy.
2. Whirl in food processor, then return to freezer until frozen solid. Remove from freezer and refrigerate for about 20 minutes to soften slightly before serving.

MAKES ABOUT 2 CUPS
APPROXIMATELY 5.0 MILLIGRAMS CHOLESTEROL
PER 1/2 CUP SERVING

◆ ◆ ◆ ◆ ◆

SHAM BRÛLÉE

▶ ▶

The traditional *crème brûlée* contains heavy cream, egg yolks, and sometimes sour cream. My mock version contains less than a third of the fat and a fraction of the cholesterol. And, it is simple to prepare.

If you like, spoon a little pureed, cooked fruit into the bottom of the cups before adding the custard, and feel free to omit the brown sugar crust. The custard is terrific with or without it.

2   *cups evaporated skim milk*
2   *tablespoons cornstarch*
¹/₄   *cup sugar*
1   *teaspoon vanilla extract*
1   *cup light sour cream*
6   *teaspoons dark brown sugar*

1. Preheat broiler.

2. In a medium saucepan, combine evaporated milk, cornstarch, sugar, and extract. Cook over low heat, stirring with a wooden spoon, for about 6 minutes or until thickened. Do not let mixture boil.

3. When thickened, let cool briefly, then combine ¹/₄ cup of the mixture with the sour cream. Gradually stir sour cream mixture into mixture in saucepan, blending well.

4. Divide mixture among six ¹/₂-cup custard cups and sprinkle tops with brown sugar. Place cups on a baking sheet

and broil about 3 inches from heat source until brown sugar is crusty. Cool briefly and serve.

SERVES 6
APPROXIMATELY 7.0 MILLIGRAMS CHOLESTEROL PER SERVING

PEACH CUSTARD
WITH ALMOND CARAMEL

▶ ▶

This delightful and unusual rendition of the traditional favorite known as *flan* in Spain or *crème caramel* in France is the just desserts for any meal.

If fresh, ripe peaches are not available, substitute fresh berries or frozen fruit.

¹/₄	cup plus 3 tablespoons sugar
4	teaspoons water
1	teaspoon almond extract
¹/₂	cup thawed frozen egg substitute
²/₃	cup whole milk
1	12-ounce can evaporated skim milk
2	teaspoons vanilla extract
2	tablespoons peach liqueur or peach nectar
6	peach halves for garnish, thinly sliced

1. Preheat oven to 300°F.

2. Mix ¹/₄ cup sugar with water in a small, heavy saucepan and cook over medium-low heat until sugar is dissolved. Increase the heat, cover the pan, and bring to a boil, swirling the pot frequently. When it bubbles, remove the lid and let mixture cook, continuing to swirl the pot and watching the mixture *very* carefully, until it begins to color (which will happen quickly). Swirl in almond extract, and when mixture is golden, remove it from the heat *immediately*. Divide the caramel among the bottoms of six ¹/₂-cup custard cups, swirl-

ing it as well as you can to coat the bottoms of the cups. Set prepared cups aside.

3. Set a kettle of water on the stove to boil. In a medium bowl, combine egg substitute with remaining 3 tablespoons sugar, stirring gently but thoroughly. When blended, gradually and gently stir in the whole milk, evaporated milk, vanilla extract, and liqueur or nectar.

4. Divide custard among the prepared cups and set the cups in a baking dish. Pour enough boiling water into the baking dish to come about ¾ of the way up the sides of the custard cups, and immediately set the baking dish in the center of the preheated oven. Bake for 1 hour and 15 minutes or until set.

5. Remove from oven and cool to room temperature, then refrigerate and chill completely. (Can be prepared one day ahead and covered well with plastic wrap.) Just before serving, run a sharp knife around the edge of the cup and invert custard and caramel onto a plate. Garnish with peach slices fanned decoratively alongside the custard.

SERVES 6
APPROXIMATELY 6.0 MILLIGRAMS CHOLESTEROL PER SERVING

INDEX

Printed in the United States
by Baker & Taylor Publisher Services